A WALK WITH PURPOSE

MICHAEL D. BECKER

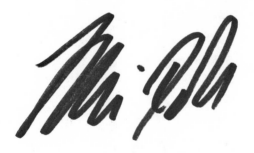

ISBN 978-1981013470 (paperback)

Cover photo by Linda Becker taken in 1998 showing Michael Becker hiking on the Iceline Trail located near Field, British Columbia in Yoho National Park.

Book website: **awalkwithpurpose.com**

This work depicts actual events in the life of the author as truthfully as recollection permits and/or can be verified by research. Occasionally, dialogue consistent with the character or nature of the person speaking has been supplemented. All persons within are actual individuals; there are no composite characters.

Second Edition

ACKNOWLEDGMENTS

This book is dedicated to my wife, love, and best friend, Lorie, who strongly encouraged me to write my story and to whom this book is dedicated. I always wanted to write a book, but in some ways, I think she wanted it even more.

Special thanks to consulting editor Alan Rinzler for his inspiration, wisdom and guidance in helping shape my story. Alan added professionalism, understanding and a clear vision with his valuable editing work.

Similarly, thank you to Brian Tedesco for editing the final manuscript and agreeing to participate in this book.

CONTENTS

Chapter One
Diagnosis

———

It was November 25th, 2015, the day before Thanksgiving, and I was in a particularly pleasant mood. Beginning my holiday a day early, I decided to work at home. As a result, I was spared the hustle and bustle of my daily commute from beautiful, rural Bucks County, Pennsylvania to New York City.

I was living a dual life, like both mice in Aesop's Fable *The Town Mouse and the Country Mouse.* During the workweek, I would enjoy the luxuries and delights of city life. Evenings and weekends were reserved for enjoying a wholesome presence in the country with the peace and serenity that go along with it. It was a pleasant balance, and I enjoyed the variety that both had to offer.

Sitting at my desk in the office adjacent to our master bedroom, I poured the last few drops of dark and intense French press coffee into my cup. Still in my pajamas, I cradled the warm mug with both hands and reflected for a moment on all of the blessings from recent weeks.

Earlier that month, I celebrated my 47th birthday and one-year anniversary at a promising new job. More recently, our wonderful neighbors, Roger and Sue Yackel, prepared a delicious Holiday feast that we enjoyed together the week prior since they were heading to Virginia to celebrate Thanksgiving with their children. Usually, we would observe Thanksgiving together if they were in town. Knowing that it's my absolute favorite meal, they went all out—turkey, mashed potatoes, stuffing, cranberries, dessert, and much, much more. Cooking an entire feast just for our benefit was one of the many acts of kindness the Yackels showed us since we first became neighbors in the autumn of 2001. They frequently surprised us with completed yard work or housework while we were away, babysat for our children and pets, and most importantly, eased our transition from Illinois to Pennsylvania by being the closest thing we had to family in the area.

After responding to some work emails, I got undressed and tiptoed gingerly up and down the cold white tiles of our bathroom floor, waiting for the shower water to heat up. Glancing at my reflection in the vast, mirrored wall above the double sink, I grabbed my abdomen with both hands, embarrassed by how much weight I'd gained recently. Weighing more than 200 pounds, even with my tall frame, was much higher than my comfort zone.

Vowing to get back into shape—*after the holidays*—I suddenly noticed something different about the right side of my neck. Placing my hand there, I could feel a lump just under my jawline that was about 3 centimeters in diameter.

Clearly, this bulge wasn't there the day before, or I would have felt it while shaving. It was a solid mass and wasn't sore at all to the touch. Putting my shower on hold, I threw my sweatpants and t-shirt back on and hurried to my office to do a quick search on the medical literature website PubMed from the U.S. National Library of Medicine.

The search results made me nervous enough to reach for the phone and call our family physician, Dr. John Sabatini. The line rang only a few times, but the wait seemed like an eternity.

"Doctor Sabatini's office..." the receptionist answered as I nearly cut her off in mid-sentence.

"Hi, this is Michael Becker. I'm a patient of Dr. Sabatini and need to make an appointment for today if at all possible."

"First, can you tell me a bit about your particular medical issue? It's the day before a holiday, and we're..."

"This is important," I interrupted, trying to keep my voice under control. "I found a rather large lump on the right side of my neck. It wasn't there yesterday."

"Okay, let me put you on hold for a moment," she said. Returning a few moments later, she continued, "Dr. Sabatini can see you at 4 o'clock if that works for you?"

"Great," I said. "That will be fine."

I hung up the phone. Rather than feeling relieved to get the appointment, I began to worry that Dr. Sabatini wanted to see me. Surely that meant it could be something serious. I was about to call my wife when my cell phone rang.

"Hey honey," Lorie said. "Just leaving school and calling to see if you want me to bring something home for lunch today?"

Since it was the day before Thanksgiving, she only had to work a half day. Lorie teaches first grade at Walt Disney Elementary School, a historic elementary school building located in Levittown, Pennsylvania. Coincidental given her love for Disney World and belief that it is indeed "the happiest place on earth." The school was dedicated in 1955 by its namesake, Walter Elias Disney himself, with each classroom based on one of Disney's characters.

"Yes, dear," I replied. "But listen, I just made an appointment with Dr. Sabatini at 4 o'clock, and I'd like you to come with me."

"What's going on?" she said, sounding alarmed. She knew that I didn't go to the doctor unless necessary, so this was a red flag.

"I found a large lump on the side of my neck before getting in the shower. It wasn't there yesterday, so I'm a bit worried."

Our two daughters, Rosie and Megan, were out with friends for the afternoon since they didn't have school. Rosie had her car and was out with a boyfriend. Megan was a few years younger and over at a friend's house. Both typical teenagers, we didn't see much of either anymore.

While waiting for Lorie to arrive home, I continued researching lateral neck masses and other relevant keywords on the Internet, looking for clues until I came across one medical journal article that contained a startling statistic:

"More than 75% of lateral neck masses in patients older than 40 years are caused by malignant tumors."[1]

———

Lorie arrived a little later with soup, sandwiches, and salad from Panera Bread, one of our frequent take-out places. As soon as she walked in from the garage, she put down the package and came over to study my neck, looking for signs of the mysterious mass.

"Oh, I see what you mean," she said with a grimace on her face. "And there was nothing there yesterday?"

"Nope," I replied. "I definitely would have noticed it while shaving."

After eating lunch together at the kitchen table, we kept ourselves busy for a few hours until it was time to leave for my appointment. When it was time, we got in our silver Toyota Highlander and headed off together to Dr. Sabatini's office. Lorie drove, and I tried to keep the conversation light. I didn't want to say anything about the statistics found on my Internet search.

It was a short 15-minute drive to Dr. Sabatini's office. As we sat in the empty exam room waiting for him to arrive, Lorie could see the look of grave concern on my face. She knew it was uncharacteristic for me to be alarmed.

"What do you think it is?" she asked.

"Cancer," I replied almost matter-of-factly.

"What??" she replied. "What kind of cancer do you think it is?"

"I don't know exactly, but I think it's a swollen lymph node—maybe lymphoma. I'm still doing some reading."

I didn't have any formal medical or scientific training but had learned quite a bit during my years both covering and working in the biotechnology sector. I didn't want to worry Lorie unnecessarily until we'd heard what Dr. Sabatini had to say. But knowing that I'm no alarmist, she wasn't prepared for my response, and her face filled immediately with concern and near tears.

Before Lorie fully processed the situation, Dr. Sabatini knocked on the exam room door and came in.

"Hello, Michael...Hi Lorie," he said. "What brings you in today?"

"This lump," I replied pointing to the right side of my neck. "I felt it this morning, and it wasn't there yesterday."

"Alright," he said, sensing the tension in the room. "Let's take a look at it."

The sweat from my palms caused the thin, white protective paper from the table to stick to my hands as he studied the growth under the bright fluorescent light of the exam room. After touching the mass gently, examining the area of my neck around it, and comparing with the other side of my neck, he sat back on his stool.

"Seems like it could be a blocked salivary gland."

"But if that were the case, wouldn't the spot be tender or painful?" I responded.

"No, not necessarily. But it could be aggravated by sour or citrus flavors that can stimulate saliva output, so try to avoid orange juice or similar beverages and foods for the next few days."

He prescribed levofloxacin, an antibiotic.

"The lump should decrease after a few days on the medication unless a stone or other obstruction is causing the blockage. If you develop severe pain or discomfort over the weekend, go the emergency room. And if there's no change then follow-up with an ear, nose, and throat (ENT) doctor on Monday."

I was feeling uneasy about the diagnosis. Could it be that simple? Or was he trying to get us through Thanksgiving festivities and not ruin our holiday?

"Do you think it could be cancer?" I blurted out.

"I wouldn't reject the possibility outright," he said, "but it would be the fifth or sixth item on the list of my considerations."

Fifth or sixth, but still on the list?

That only fueled our anxiety. Lorie and I would have felt much better if cancer was significantly lower on his list, or better yet, not included at all. But my research had already shown that such an exclusion was highly unlikely.

We returned home, our heads spinning with endless questions and little concrete information. All we could do is wait and see if the lump responded to the antibiotic.

With the exception that cancer was on the list of considerations, we relayed Dr. Sabatini's encouraging blocked salivary gland prognosis to Rosie and Megan, downplaying that there was any reason for concern. However, knowing it was a rare occasion that I would see the doctor, they still found it odd.

————

I checked every morning before showering, but there was no change in the size or density of the lump on my neck over the weekend, despite being on the antibiotic. Based on more extensive online research, I had already narrowed my self-diagnosis to head and neck cancer.

I didn't have an established relationship with an ENT physician. Lorie, on the other hand, battled constant sinus infections and had her otolaryngologist, Dr. John Gallagher, on speed dial. On my behalf, she phoned Bucks ENT Associates in Langhorne, Pennsylvania to try and book an appointment for me on Monday, November 30th, but Dr. Gallagher wasn't available. Knowing time was of the essence; she instead scheduled for the following day with one of his colleagues, Dr. Jeffrey Briglia.

Since the appointment wasn't until early Tuesday afternoon, I went to work in New York for a half day in the morning. Lorie couldn't take the afternoon off work to accompany me, as her school district's policy prohibited taking leave following a holiday.

"So, what brings you here today, Michael?" Dr. Briglia asked, smiling.

As if to say "duh," I pointed directly to the protruding bump on my neck and explained my story.

"I found this lump the morning before Thanksgiving Day and saw my family physician, who suspected an infection and put me on an antibiotic. Despite several days of treatment, there's been no reduction in size. I'm concerned that it's likely cancer."

His smile quickly diminished.

"There are many other possibilities besides malignancy for this lump, Michael. It could simply be a cyst or even a..."

"I know, but the odds are against it," I interrupted him. "I'm not a doctor, but I've been around the biotechnology industry long enough to pick up a few things. In reading some medical journals, I came across the fact that more than 75 percent of lateral neck masses in patients over forty are caused by malignant tumors."

"I see, well..." he was taken aback, or perhaps more likely offended, viewing me merely as another patient trying to play Dr. Google. I couldn't tell but plowed on.

"I'm not interested in false hope or encouragement," I said. "If it is cancer, I'd rather know sooner than later so that I can begin exploring treatment options as soon as possible."

I paused.

Dr. Briglia didn't say anything for a while, gathering his thoughts, I assumed, then spoke.

"Alright, then. Let's take a closer look and see what's going on."

"Excellent," I said, feeling confident that I had flexed enough of my medical knowledge to establish a more collegial relationship with him.

His first diagnostic approach was a flexible endoscopy procedure.

"I'm going to insert a thin, lighted tube with a camera through your nasal cavity," he explained, "so we can examine hard-to-see areas such as the larynx and behind the nose."

With the flip of a switch, Dr. Briglia started a small air compressor unit that powered the spray of local anesthesia ("lidocaine," he told me) into each of my nostrils. This way, I wouldn't feel discomfort or gag as the thin tube snaked its way up my nose, then curved back down towards my throat. I grimaced from the bitter, medicinal taste entering my mouth as the lidocaine drained down my sinuses and into my throat. Dr. Briglia paused for a while to allow the anesthetic to work, then proceeded to insert the thin tube up my right nostril gently. I started to watch the live view from the tiny camera on the nearby computer monitor.

"Nothing suspicious looking here," he said after retracting the camera. "I'd like to order a CT scan to see inside the lump and get a better sense of what is going on."

Nothing suspicious? Was I wrong and it wasn't cancer? He handed me a few tissues to clean up my runny nose after the procedure and then escorted me out to the reception area to get an order for the CT.

————

The CT, or computed tomography, imaging procedure was scheduled for late afternoon on December 2nd, 2015 at St.

15

Mary's Medical Center, which is also close to our home. It was after school got out, so Lorie was able to come with me this time.

After navigating the maze of fluorescent corridors at St. Mary's, we arrived at the radiology department. I put my name on the sign-in sheet, and we found two seats together in the crowded waiting area.

It wasn't long before the door to the CT room opened, and a nurse called my name. Once through the door, I noticed the room was extremely light and bright, but more importantly, very cold. From my experience, I knew CT scanners needed to be kept chilly during operation. What I didn't expect was a room so frosty that you could safely store meat.

I was given a paper gown and instructed to change. The nurse returned and explained the CT procedure would involve an intravenous infusion of an iodinated contrast agent, sometimes referred to as "dye." The dye is used to make specific organs, blood vessels and tissue types "stand out" with more image contrast to show the presence of disease or injury.

"Any history of allergies, diabetes, asthma, a heart condition, kidney problems, or thyroid conditions?" the nurse asked.

"Nope."

"Excellent," she replied and began inserting a needle into a vein in my left forearm, which was then held in place with tape. A clear, thin tube connected my vein to the contrast agent. "You may feel a warm or hot flushed sensation during the actual injection of the dye and a metallic taste in the mouth, which usually lasts less than a minute or so. Both are perfectly normal and no need for concern."

The words did nothing to alleviate my more significant fear since I knew more dangerous allergic reactions associated with contrast agents, although quite rare, include breathing difficulty, swelling of the throat, or other parts of the body that could be more serious if not treated immediately.

"I'll be in the other room monitoring you during the procedure the entire time, so if you need anything ask," she said as she exited the room.

I'm not usually claustrophobic, but the big white enamel tube they slid me into and the whirring sound the machine made as it began spinning around made me uneasy. Over the intercom, the nurse provided periodic updates, such as the amount of time remaining and when the infusion of the contrast agent would begin.

Finally, it was over. I was taken out of the submarine and got dressed. Dr. Briglia had instructed me to get a CD-ROM with the results of the CT scan right after the procedure to bring with me to my follow-up appointment the next day. Lorie and I stopped by a nearby window afterward and picked-up the disk.

During my tenure working at local biotechnology company Cytogen Corporation, I had seen my share of radiology reports and images—especially concerning cancer and lymph nodes. At one point, the company had licensed marketing rights to a unique contrast agent being developed by Advanced Magnetics, Inc. to help physicians distinguish between cancerous and non-cancerous lymph nodes using magnetic resonance imaging (MRI). Unfortunately, the investigational product never received marketing approval from the Food and Drug Administration (FDA) and development was eventually discontinued.

When I arrived home, I attempted to load the CD on my Mac computer. Unfortunately, the software for viewing the CT images only worked on Windows computers. I'd have to wait for my ENT appointment for the results.

———

Lorie took a half-day at work so that she could join me the next afternoon for my follow-up ENT appointment. After calling my name, we were both escorted back to the exam room. Dr. Briglia entered after a few minutes, and I handed him the CD from the prior day's CT scan. He took the disc and exited the room to retrieve a laptop computer for viewing.

When he returned with the computer, it took forever for the images to load from the CD due to the volume and resolution of the files.

"Can we go over the radiology report while we're waiting?" I asked impatiently.

Dr. Briglia was still fiddling with his computer and appeared not to hear from me.

"Dr. Briglia?" I said, about to ask again, but he remained focused on getting the images to appear on the computer screen.

So much for establishing a collegial relationship. His actions not only irritated me but also heightened my fear that he'd already read the radiologist's report and that it must contain some bad news.

When the images finally materialized on the computer screen, Dr. Briglia scrolled through to the relevant cross-section images where the suspicious neck mass resided.

As soon as the images popped up on the screen, I knew the result. There it was—the classic presentation of an enlarged lymph node infiltrated by cancer. Normal lymph nodes are tiny and can be hard to find, but when there's infection, inflammation, or cancer, the nodes can get larger. Lymph nodes greater than one centimeter in diameter are deemed suspicious—and mine measured more than 4 centimeters on its longest axis. Not only that, the enlarged node had a dark necrotic core like a cross-section of a jelly doughnut, with the thin, bright outer layer encasing a sea of cellular debris. This pattern of central lymph node necrosis has been reported to carry nearly 100 percent accuracy in predicting the presence of metastatic disease.[2] My stomach sank.

"Yup, sure looks like a lymph node invaded by cancer," I said, anything but proud that my initial self-diagnosis of cancer was looking accurate.

"It does look suspicious," he agreed, "but it could still be something benign. The only way to know for sure is to take the next step in the process."

"A biopsy?"

"Right," he said. "We'll do a fine needle aspiration, right now and right here."

After assembling a series of glass microscope slides on the counter, he injected the area on my neck with lidocaine before using a more substantial syringe to extract material from inside the suspicious lymph node. Such biopsies can be a hit-or-miss procedure, as success requires removing enough living cancer cells from among the dead cells at the necrotic center of the lymph node.

I felt the sharp stick of the needle from the anesthetic injection, followed by a slight burning sensation before the right side of my neck started going numb. I looked over at Lorie, who was seated on a chair across the exam room. She could tell how bad the initial injection hurt from the expression on my face and looked at me with great sympathy.

I didn't feel the second needle stick as Dr. Briglia carefully probed the mass and collected material using a syringe. Finally, he released a small portion of the syringe contents onto each glass slide, placing a small square on top to seal each one. Then he packed the slides into a kit in preparation for being shipped to an external pathology lab for analysis.

"It takes about a week for results to come back," he announced.

Great. More waiting, I thought to myself.

Six days later, I was at my desk in New York City. My employer at the time, Relmada Therapeutics, had moved to a temporary office near Third Avenue and 47th Street over the summer while work was being completed at the company's new corporate headquarters a few blocks away. Since it was temporary space, we rented four offices with anywhere from two to four people in each one, grouped by job function. Relmada's CEO, Sergio Traversa, hired me as senior vice president of finance and corporate development about a year before. I shared an office with Christine Berni-Silverstein, director of investor relations, who'd been hired around the same time. We focused the majority of our efforts on investor relations and capital raising activities, so it made sense to pair us together. Neither of us had yet seen the new headquarters, which wouldn't be ready until late December.

A little before lunchtime, my cell phone rang. Looking at the caller ID, I knew it was the ENT with the biopsy results. I jumped out of my seat to take the call in a vacant conference room nearby, which would be more private.

"Hello, Dr. Briglia," I said nervously.

Unlike prior pussy-footing around with a lot of hedging concerning the possible diagnosis, the doctor spoke quickly and frankly this time.

"I'm sorry to say that the biopsy confirmed the presence of squamous cell carcinoma, or cancer, in the lymph node."

Even though I already knew the diagnosis in my heart, hearing him say the word cancer was disheartening. Most of my career focused on companies working in the cancer segment of the biotechnology industry, but none of that experience prepared me for my diagnosis.

"Can you please email me a copy of the cytology report?" I inquired after we'd discussed the laboratory results in greater detail.

"Um, sure...I guess we can do that," he replied, seeming a bit puzzled. But I knew that a copy of the report would be helpful as I began researching my disease and began outreach to relevant medical contacts.

Dr. Briglia informed me that the next step would be a positron emission tomography, or PET, functional imaging procedure used to observe metabolic processes in the body—the use of sugar in particular. This nuclear medicine imaging procedure uses fludeoxyglucose (FDG), a radioactive analogue of glucose, or sugar, to highlight metabolic activity corresponding with abnormally high glucose uptake in particular tissue, which includes organs like the brain and liver, but, more importantly, cancer, which uses sugar to a much more significant degree than healthy cells or tissue. Finding areas of high glucose uptake where it isn't usually expected can be associated with malignancy.

Knowing that the lymph node in my neck was cancerous, it would be expected to show up on the PET scan. More importantly, other locations of cancer should also be visible, which would help identify where the disease originated and where else it had spread.

In general, cancer can appear in the lymph nodes in one of two ways: either it originates there, or it can spread there from somewhere else. Cancer that begins in the lymph nodes is called lymphoma. More often, however, disease starts someplace else and then spreads to lymph nodes. That's why we needed a PET scan to identify the starting location and extent of spread, or metastatic disease.

After finishing with Dr. Briglia, I phoned Lorie's cell phone immediately, as promised.

"Can you talk?" I asked.

"Just for a minute. The kids are at special, and I need to pick them up soon."

"The results were as I expected," I said. "I've got cancer."

"I *so* wanted you to be wrong this time," she gasped.

"I know. Me too. I'm so sorry, honey..."

"No... no..." She choked up and then started to sob. For as much as I was convinced from the start that I had cancer, Lorie is an eternal optimist and refused to believe for a moment that the lump was anything but benign. That is, until now.

"We'll talk more tonight when I get home from work," I said.

"Okay," she said in a muffled voice. "I have to go get my kids."

"Love you."

"Love you too...bye."

We both hung up.

I stood silently and alone in the conference room staring out the window to the vast metropolis below. *Why me? Why now?* I thought as a few isolated tears streamed down my cheeks.

After trying to compose myself for a minute, I returned to my office. I knew that I wouldn't be able to disguise my concern over the news, so I opted to inform my colleague of the diagnosis.

"Christine," I said.

She looked up from her computer screen.

"What is it, Michael? You look upset."

"Right," I said. "Listen, I just got the biopsy results, and they confirm it is cancer."

"Oh no, Michael. I'm so sorry to hear that!"

"I know it's unfair to dump this on you right now, but..."

"Not at all. Is there anything I can do?"

"Thanks, but I'm still processing it all. The first thing that I'm going to do is talk to some medical oncologists that I know and see what they say about available treatment options."

"Listen," she said softly but sternly, "I vow to keep any and all negativity out of this office." She put up her right hand as if taking an oath. "You're going to beat this, and there will only be positive vibes in our office from this moment on."

I felt horrible dropping the news on Christine. She was still recovering from the devastating loss of a good friend, Lauren Del Vecchio-Zaleski, due to a chronic illness called scleroderma with an overlap of lupus and fibromyalgia. These autoimmune diseases affected her heart, causing it to be covered in scar tissue. Lauren had taken her last breath on July 19th, 2013.

After a short while, an email arrived from Dr. Briglia's office with the cytology report. It was a simple, one-page document with my personal information at the top, a paragraph of dense medical terminology in the middle, and a few photomicrographs of the biopsy specimens. One line, however, put it quite plainly:

Diagnosis—Right neck: Poorly differentiated squamous cell carcinoma

Cancers that are known collectively as head and neck cancers usually begin in the squamous cells that line the moist, mucosal surfaces inside the head and neck. The fact that my cancer cells were "poorly differentiated" meant that they looked very different from the cells from which they arose. In general, well-differentiated tumors behave better than poorly differentiated tumors.

By late morning I also spoke with Sergio to let him know about my diagnosis.

"Oh my, I'm so sorry to hear that," he said with his strong Italian accent. "Listen, take off whenever you need for doctor appointments, treatments, whatever. Consider your schedule here completely flexible. Getting you back to good health is the top priority."

Needing some time to reflect on the diagnosis, I told him I'd leave work early that afternoon.

———

When I arrived home that evening, Lorie and I embraced tightly for a long time. The emotions stored up throughout the day needed a release. We sobbed together.

After drying our tears, we called the girls down from upstairs to have a family meeting so that we could break the news to them. They were both in high school at the time, so we felt that they were old enough to receive the news unvarnished. That being said, I thought it was also imperative for them to have hope.

We all sat down on the large, brown leather sectional couch. Lorie and I sat next to each other; Rosie and Megan sat across from us.

"As you both know," I began, "your mother and I have been expecting the results of my biopsy, which came today. Unfortunately, the diagnosis is cancer."

Both girls sat almost motionless amid the silence that followed. Their eyes started to water.

"Wait," I said trying to halt the inevitable, visceral reaction. "I know cancer is a terrifying word that conjures visions of doom and gloom, but there have been a lot of advances regarding treatment, especially in the area of cancer immunotherapy. More and more, cancer is becoming a chronic illness that can be managed, not dissimilar to other diseases, such as diabetes."

"And you know your father is a smart man," Lorie interceded. "With his biotechnology experience and industry contacts, you can count on him to do everything he can to beat this thing. Right?"

The girls hesitantly nodded in agreement.

"So, let's keep it positive," Lorie went on, trying hard to embody the words herself.

Despite remaining upbeat and keeping my emotions hidden, no one likes uncertainty, and there was plenty of that to go around. What treatments were available? How quickly would my quality of life diminish? Most importantly, how much time did I have left?

Towards the end of the brief discussion, amid the tears and silence, both girls came over and gave me a long hug. During the embrace, I glanced across the room at Gracie, our German Shepherd. Suddenly, it occurred to me that in the weeks and months before my cancer diagnosis, she spent an unusual amount of time with her nose very close to my face and the right side of my neck, sniffing intently. She's a sweet pup, so we figured she was being affectionate and didn't think much of it at the time. But studies from France to California to Italy have concluded that dogs really can detect the smell of cancer, and I wondered if that helped explain her unusual actions.

———

It had been a little over two-weeks since I first discovered the lump on my neck. While it had appeared overnight, cancer had probably been there for quite some time. As a result, I felt an overwhelming sense of urgency to begin treatment—anything to help reverse the current course. I started researching experts in the area of head and neck cancer.

Fortunately, throughout my career, I had forged several close relationships with key opinion leaders in the fields of both oncology and immunology. Most of them concentrated in the area of prostate cancer since that was the primary disease focus of Cytogen Corporation, where I served as CEO from 2002-2007. Nevertheless, I emailed Susan Slovin, M.D., Ph.D., a medical oncologist at Memorial Sloan-Kettering Cancer Center (MSKCC) with expertise in prostate cancer, clinical immunology, and other genitourinary malignancies, such as bladder cancer.

I always had tremendous respect for Dr. Slovin. She was an expert in her field and never afraid to speak her mind or offer a contrarian opinion. She could be blunt, which was an attribute of hers I much appreciated—especially at times like this. She also had a fabulous sense of humor and referred to me as "Young'n" given my rise to CEO at an early age.

Early the next morning, I wrote Dr. Slovin an email.

"When you have a few moments, I need to know if there is a squamous cell carcinoma expert you can direct me to at MSKCC. I was hoping it was nothing a week ago, but pathology confirmed today."

She replied quickly and with her typical direct but entertaining fashion.

"Sorry to hear but squamous of what? Skin, lung, pecker????"

Good grief, could I have cancer of the penis? I thought for a second.

"Happy to share any of the reports (pathology, CT scan, etc.)," I quickly typed back, "but at this point 4cm lymph node in neck, so they are speculating oral cancer. Getting a full body PET next to find out where the primary tumor is, which will answer a lot of questions, although I hear sometimes the primary is difficult to find."

"All fixable," she replied. "Dr. David Pfister is great here. His office number is on the website. We need the actual biopsy slides. Let's get going. No time for tears or self-pity."

I wasted no time and found Dr. Pfister's contact information on the Internet. After speaking with his office, I replied back to Dr. Slovin.

"They took all my info, asked for copies of radiology report and pathology report, which I am emailing to them next. They need the PET scan results before sending to Dr.

Pfister. I assume to make sure it isn't some other cancer that he doesn't handle. Anyway, hoping to get PET scan done tomorrow or Friday at the latest."

"Get the PET scan done ASAP and the slides. Use my name. It inspires fear!!!" she concluded half-jokingly.

David Pfister, M.D. is a medical oncologist at MSKCC specializing in head and neck malignancies including tumors of the mouth, throat, thyroid, salivary glands, and skin. It didn't take me long to figure out that this was a great fit, as he was part of the multidisciplinary team at MSKCC that cured actor Michael Douglas, who received a diagnosis of stage IV oropharyngeal cancer in 2010.

Thanks to Dr. Slovin, I was able to schedule the first available appointment with Dr. Pfister, which was early in the morning on Christmas Eve. I suspect she worked behind-the-scenes to get me in before the next regular slot.

I wanted to know my prognosis and therapeutic options, but more importantly, I wanted to begin treatment. Since Thanksgiving, I spent every day looking in the mirror and seeing a large mass on the right side of my neck. Taunting me, it was a constant visual reminder of the disease, and I wanted it gone. Immediately.

———

My PET scan was scheduled at St. Mary's Medical Center. Having the CT scan done there a little over a week ago, I wasn't overly apprehensive about the PET scan. It was a late morning appointment, so the most significant issue for me was being unable to drink my usual pot of coffee, or anything else other than water until after the procedure.

Rosie had the day off from school, so she was able to accompany me for the PET scan. She kept herself entertained on her iPhone in the waiting area, while a nurse brought me back to a room where the radioactive FDG injection was administered. Following the dose, I had to wait an hour for the drug to circulate before being scanned. This procedure was much longer than the first CT scan and took around two hours total.

"Sorry you had to wait long," I said to Rosie upon returning to the waiting area.

"No problem," she replied. "Some woman from a local church came around and handed out these cute little bags full of snacks and a bottle of water to everyone in the waiting area. Wasn't that nice of them?"

"Wow, yes—that was very kind. Which reminds me, let's stop by the cafeteria and get me a cup of coffee to go."

We arrived back home. By now, I was aware that St. Mary's Medical Center offered an online patient portal that provided access to radiology reports from imaging studies performed there. By mid-afternoon that same day I was able to read the full text of the radiology report online, which suggested that cancer originated in my right tonsil and then escaped, spreading to nearby lymph nodes in my neck.

The formal diagnosis was oropharyngeal cancer, a disease in which malignant cells form in the tissue of oropharynx—the middle part of the throat that includes the base of the tongue, the tonsils, the soft palate, and the walls of the pharynx.

In plain English, I had advanced head and neck cancer.

My background in oncology was both a blessing and a curse. I knew that "staging" describes the severity of a person's cancer based on the size and reach of the original, primary tumor, and whether or not cancer has spread in the body. Staging is essential for several reasons, including helping the doctor plan appropriate treatment and estimating a patient's prognosis, which is the chance of recovery. Given the fact that my high-grade cancer originated in the right tonsil and had already spread from this primary site to the regional lymph nodes on the right side of my neck, I realized that my prognosis was quite poor.

Doctors combine the staging criteria for tumor (T), lymph node (N), and metastasis (M), also known as TNM, to determine the stage of disease for each person. Most cancers have four stages: stages I to IV. The higher the number, the larger the cancer tumor and the more it has spread. Applying the TNM criteria for oral and oropharyngeal cancer that I found through my online research, I concluded that I had stage IV disease since the enlarged lymph node measured more than 3 centimeters and more than one lymph node was invaded according to the PET scan and accompanying radiology report.

Being curious by nature, I continued learning as much as I could about oropharyngeal cancer and its treatment by reading medical journals and various articles. I even came across the transcript of a talk by actor and producer Michael Douglas, who was speaking at a prestigious cancer conference about his experience with stage IV oropharyngeal cancer.

Douglas credited his favorable outcome to the team at MSKCC, which included Dr. Pfister. In the article, he described his seven weeks of radiation and chemotherapy as "very accurately mapped to the seven cycles of hell, and each week I sank a little lower, and I felt a lot worse."

Finding information about my particular cancer wasn't easy, as head and neck cancers are relatively rare. According to the American Cancer Society, approximately 65,000 men and women in this country were diagnosed with head and neck cancers in 2017.

Sensing an unmet need, I decided to start a blog chronicling my cancer journey. I hoped that some of the content might be a helpful resource for others dealing with head and neck cancer. It would be an efficient vehicle to keep family and friends updated about my progress. By sharing my experience freely, I also wanted to create greater awareness for the disease and its impact.

———

Patience has never been my strong suit, so waiting over a week for an initial consultation with Dr. Pfister didn't sit well with me. Little did I know that it could take weeks or longer to see a physician of his caliber.

Adding to my anxiety was the fact that the cervical lymph node on my neck was both visible and palpable. I was reminded of the disease every time I looked in the mirror, shaved, or placed my hand on the area. As a result, I was keen to get started with treatment despite any associated side effects. I just wanted it gone—now! Christmas day would be exactly one month since I first discovered the suspicious growth and I couldn't help but feel that cancer was being given too much time to grow and spread.

Following a "formal" cancer diagnoses, which itself can take weeks waiting for biopsy and imaging results, I mistakenly envisioned that a S.W.A.T. team of physicians rushed in to start treatment. In reality, it can take weeks to schedule appointments with some doctors—especially those in high demand. Also, for some procedures, such as radiation therapy, the process also involves complex treatment planning to deliver a customized dose of radiation to the tumor and spare healthy tissue. Doing so requires getting fitted for a unique reinforced thermoplastic mask to hold the patient steady within a few millimeters for consistency each day during the seven-week therapy.

Knowing it never hurts to get a second opinion, and in my desperation to try and accelerate the process, I started calling local oncologists to try and schedule an appointment.

The first phone call was to nearby University of Pennsylvania (UPenn), where the receptionist seemed somewhat perplexed by my request.

"It's usually a physician who refers patients to our center," she said. "How do you know you have cancer?"

"I read both the radiology and pathology reports," I replied.

After a few minutes on hold, an appointment with a medical oncologist was scheduled for mid-December; precisely one week before my initial visit with Dr. Pfister at MSKCC.

I had no idea what to expect when Lorie and I arrived at UPenn for the appointment. The waiting area was crowded with patients at various stages in their disease, ranging from newly diagnosed (me) to patients who had cancer for a long time. Some of the patients looked fine, but others seemed quite weary from their battle—tired, frail, often tethered to IV poles, most of them expressionless.

I couldn't help but wonder which of this cast of characters would I identify most in the coming months? I had spent most of my career as an outsider to the oncology community, but now I was on the front lines. Just the latest soldier enlisted to fight a common enemy. It was sobering.

While I had already read the radiology report from my recent PET scan, I couldn't view the actual images on the CD from my Mac computer at home. Fortunately, during the appointment at UPenn, the medical oncologist, Dr. Joshua Bauml, put them up on a computer screen in his office. For the first time since my diagnosis, Lorie and I finally saw the "enemy"—the bright, yellow/orange glowing areas in the PET images that represented cancer. One such spot was my tonsil, where the disease originated, and the other was the enlarged lymph node in my neck, where it had spread. Both locations were on the right side of my body.

"You have stage IV oropharyngeal, or head and neck, cancer," he stated. "The location of the malignant lymph node near the carotid artery could make surgery difficult, but that can be discussed at our next multidisciplinary tumor board. The combination of chemotherapy and radiation (chemoradiation) would be the most likely initial treatment."

In this scenario, he explained to us, chemotherapy (cisplatin) would be primarily used to make the cancer cells more susceptible to the lethal effects of the accompanying radiation treatment in addition to killing cancer cells itself.

"The whole course of therapy would span 6-7 weeks. Daily radiation treatment Monday through Friday in addition to three cycles of chemotherapy spread evenly throughout. Since it does not appear that cancer has spread below the collarbone, the goal of the treatment would be curative," he said reassuringly.

There was no sugar coating the side effects of treatment, however, which Dr. Bauml told us would start to kick in around week four and beyond. The toxicities from radiation exposure are cumulative and would get worse with each treatment.

"It's no picnic," he said openly. "But there's a good chance that the treatment could be effective. So, I hope that possibility will help you get through it."

The next step was to meet with a radiation oncologist and discuss various options, such as intensity-modulated radiation therapy or IMRT. IMRT is an advanced mode of high-precision radiotherapy that uses computer-controlled delivery of precise radiation doses to a malignant tumor or specific areas within the tumor. Doing so helps minimize damage to surrounding healthy tissue and organs.

UPenn, however, is one of the few centers in the region also to offer newer "proton therapy." In this process, a proton beam conforms to the shape of a tumor with greater precision while sparing nearby healthy tissues and organs. Dr. Bauml said proton therapy could be an option for me depending on feedback from the radiation oncologist at a subsequent visit.

"One of the main side effects from cisplatin includes hearing loss," Dr. Bauml told us, "which is why you need to schedule a hearing test to get a baseline reading."

"*What?*" I replied as though I had trouble hearing him. Lorie rolled her eyes, having listened to my routine a thousand times.

He laughed, not having heard the witticism before. Most people facing a cancer diagnosis don't joke around, but I've always used humor as a defense mechanism. Dr. Bauml continued, "If there were any issues with hearing loss before therapy, it could rule out the use of cisplatin, and we have other chemotherapies that would be considered."

"Radiation therapy can also lead to mouth sores and dental problems," he added. By this time, Lorie and I were exhausted, trying to remember all these potential obstacles and options. "This means you'll also meet with a dentist at UPenn. Best case is that all of these meetings can be coordinated on the same day as part of the follow-up appointment with the radiation oncologist."

"How quickly do you think I can get started with the treatment?" I asked.

"I would hope to begin therapy within the first few weeks of January," he concluded.

Assuming that the treatment slipped into the third week of January, it would be precisely two months since discovering the lump on my neck before starting treatment. My frustration was growing with intensity each passing day.

On December 23rd, 2015, Lorie, Rosie, Megan, and I drove to New York City to stay overnight at the DoubleTree by Hilton Hotel ahead of my appointment the next morning to discuss my case with Dr. Pfister at MSKCC. The hotel was located at Lexington Avenue and 51st Street in the heart of Midtown Manhattan's fashionable East Side. Lorie and I were in one room, with Rosie and Megan sharing a room directly across the hall.

Before adjourning to our room for the evening, Lorie and I stopped at the lobby bar for a nightcap. Forgoing my usual red wine consumption wasn't an option, especially given everything going on. The lounge was quite crowded, but we found two seats together at the bar.

"Where are you leaning towards for treatment," Lorie asked me. "Here or University of Pennsylvania?"

"UPenn," I said after taking a large sip of wine. "Largely because they're moving faster. But I'm also worried about the daily commute for both treatment and work. UPenn is a little closer to home but less convenient for getting to New York for work after treatment. MSKCC is geographically more desirable, as it would only be a taxi or subway ride back to the office."

"That's assuming, of course, that you feel okay to go to work after treatment," she said. "Why don't we wait until we hear what Dr. Pfister has to say before making a firm decision."

"You're right, of course. I'm anxious to get treatment started."

"I know you are. So am I."

I signaled to the bartender for another glass of wine to take with me back to the room. After paying the bill, we headed back upstairs to check on the girls before bed.

The next morning, Rosie and Megan stayed back at the hotel for some extra sleep as Lorie and I arrived at Dr. Pfister's office on 64th Street between Second and Third Avenues. We checked in with the receptionist and then sat quietly together in the waiting area before being escorted to an exam room.

Dr. Pfister's tall, slender frame made quite an impression as he entered the room. After the requisite introductions, he mentioned hearing from Dr. Slovin, and we discussed pleasantries about my biotechnology background and how she and I had first met.

"Look, there's little ambiguity regarding your diagnosis," he said returning to the matter at hand. "You have Stage IV oropharyngeal cancer. The good news, if there is such a thing, is that the tumor appears to be positive for human papillomavirus, or HPV. Such cancers tend to respond better to chemoradiation than their HPV-negative counterparts. We've had many patients do quite well."

His calm, confident presence and encouraging words were a welcome departure from the negativity churning in my mind. However, the serenity lasted only a few moments before Dr. Pfister informed me that another biopsy might be required to confirm the HPV status, but that he'd double-check to see if the ENT's biopsy would suffice. Additionally, he wanted to do another flexible endoscopy procedure to view the tonsils while I was there.

After the endoscopy procedure, Dr. Pfister continued with a physical exam of my neck area.

"The enlarged cervical lymph node seems tethered in its location," he said after trying to move the lump around with his fingers, "which could mean that the cancer is spreading outside of the node, what we call an extracapsular invasion."

Next, we discussed potential treatments along with their pros and cons. Dr. Pfister mentioned chemoradiation; same as the UPenn oncologist. But the conversation shifted to possible clinical trials, and Dr. Pfister said one, in particular, is exploring an alternative to chemotherapy and may have fewer side effects. In the study, the chemotherapy agent (cisplatin) is replaced by Erbitux® (cetuximab)—another FDA approved agent for treating head and neck cancer. Erbitux is a type of biological therapy called a monoclonal antibody that blocks the epidermal growth factor receptor (EGFR) found on both normal and tumor cells. But the study also adds an investigational agent BYL719, which is an inhibitor of PI3K, an enzyme that fuels the growth of several types of cancer.

Once again, I appreciated that after spending so many years leading a few small, oncology-focused biotechnology companies developing immunotherapies, radiopharmaceutical agents, and supportive care oncology products, I was able to utilize that experience, knowledge, and network to make informed treatment decisions. Like driving on a familiar road, I continually saw landmarks and signs that I knew quite well from my time in the industry.

While the streets may have been familiar, I was still faced with difficult decisions at some of the crossroads. For instance, the chemotherapy commonly used in head and neck cancer patients is cisplatin, which was first approved for use in testicular and ovarian cancers back in 1978.[3] Biologic agents and inhibitors of the PI3K pathway were newer and potentially more exciting than an old chemotherapy drug. However, trading the proven results with cisplatin for "potentially" similar efficacy with lower side effects from the investigational combination was a difficult decision.

I decided to stick with traditional cisplatin for a variety of reasons. First, radiation therapy would be included regardless of whether I opted for cisplatin or the investigational Erbitux/BYL719 combination. And radiation is the driving force for both treatment efficacy *and* debilitating side effects. Most of cisplatin's side effects, such as nausea, constipation, kidney damage, and other issues, could be managed with medication and hydration. Second, cisplatin has been around for decades and appears to be the gold standard in combination with radiation for Stage IV head and neck cancer. It was hard to argue with the significant clinical data supporting its use to date. Finally, in the unfortunate event that chemoradiation wasn't curative, I could always explore investigational treatments as a next step.

"Okay, Dr. Pfister," I said. "Let's go ahead with chemoradiation. The faster, the better."

I was happy about the decision, and so was Lorie, who had favored MSKCC in the first place.

After the visit with Dr. Pfister, Lorie and I went back to have lunch with Rosie and Megan. It was unseasonably warm that day—around 70 degrees Fahrenheit. We took advantage of the weather to dine al fresco at Dos Caminos, a Mexican restaurant that was close to the hotel and not far from my office.

"I was here once before with some colleagues," I said as everyone glanced at their menus, "they have delicious guacamole."

"That sounds nice. You know how I love good guacamole," said Lorie with a smile, as we attempted to keep the mood light with small talk.

Neither of us had much of an appetite, but we tried to put on a good show for the sake of Rosie and Megan. I'm not sure which was more surreal; dining al fresco in the middle of winter in New York, or putting the distractions of the moment behind us—if only for the short duration of a meal.

By the time the check had arrived, the mood was somber again. No one felt motivated to walk around the city and look at the holiday decorations or store windows. We headed back home to Pennsylvania.

Dr. Pfister's office helped expedite subsequent appointments with one of MSKCC's radiation oncologists, Dr. Nancy Lee, who is vice-chair in their department of radiation oncology, experimental therapeutics, along with one of their surgeons, Dr. Benjamin Roman, to get their perspectives on relevant treatment options.

I knew that both chemoradiation and surgery were "potentially" curative treatment options for me. During the separate appointments with these two doctors, I learned about some of the differences regarding side effects and maintaining a good quality of life going forward.

In my particular case, based on the stage and extent of disease, a surgeon could theoretically remove the tonsils, enlarged lymph node, and surrounding soft tissue with the hope of getting all the cancer. Under the "clean margins" scenario, I could be spared chemotherapy and its toxicities and just go through radiation therapy as a next step.

If the surgical procedure didn't result in clean margins, however, then chemotherapy would be included along with the radiation therapy, and the surgery would have been somewhat pointless. More importantly, it would expose me to potentially severe side effects—such as difficulties in speech, swallowing, and other issues due to the apparent spread of cancer to my soft palate.

Armed with this insight, it was clear that surgery was an unattractive option, and Drs. Lee and Roman both confirmed the plan to move forward solely with chemoradiation. Baby steps, but it was nice to rule out surgery as a treatment option and focus on chemoradiation. The closest procedure I ever had to an operation was getting my wisdom teeth removed as a teenager. For some reason, the thought of going under the knife always terrified me, so I was happy to keep my surgery-free track record intact.

———

One of Lorie's favorite paintings hangs in the Art Institute of Chicago—A Sunday Afternoon on the Island of La Grande Jatte, by Georges Seurat. Seurat was the French post-Impressionist, who, working with Paul Signac, developed a radical new style of painting called "pointillism."

The pointillism technique uses small, distinct dots of color applied in patterns that can be seen up close. Looking at such a painting from a distance, our eyes and brains blend all of the dots of color into a fuller range of tones that form a recognizable image.

My initial meeting with the radiation oncology team at MSKCC on January 3rd, 2016, reminded me of pointillism. Before the visit, I saw the complete picture from afar—it would be 6-7 weeks of treatment and the associated side effects, but there was the prospect of being cancer-free by the end. After the meeting, however, I started seeing many individual dots of color that represented my treatment.

For example, on the first day, they created the "mask" that prevents any movement of my head and shoulders, keeping me in the same place for my daily radiation treatment. For the fitting, technicians placed a slightly hot, pliable material on my face, neck, and shoulders, which they quickly manipulated to fit the contour of my body before solidifying. Unlike the older generation masks, there was now a cutout for the patient's eyes, nose, and mouth, but total coverage of the jaw largely prevents you from speaking or opening your mouth. For each day's radiation course, the resulting mask is bolted to the treatment table—completely immobilizing you from the shoulders on up.

Frankly, the mask was terrifying! I underwent three separate imaging procedures in the afternoon (MRI, CT, and PET), and each one involved wearing the mask for about 30 minutes. Each time I was rolled into the imaging tube, I couldn't help but think, *what happens if I start coughing, sneezing, or even choking?* With my jaw and head immobilized, I wouldn't be able to do much. Trying to get past that fear, I quickly realized that I'd better get used to it. Wearing the mask would become a daily routine for the next 6-7 weeks. Fortunately, the IMRT treatment sessions were much shorter than the imaging procedures—lasting only about 10-minutes or so.

The side effects of radiation therapy were another one of the individual dots of color that came into focus as I looked more closely at my treatment "image." For instance, I lost count of how many physicians and nurses told me to "bulk up" now before starting therapy.

"Gain at least ten pounds," one nurse had told me. "In a few weeks, you might start developing oral mucositis and dry mouth from the radiation, and it'll be tough for you to chew, or swallow," said another. "You may get pretty tired, too."

Coincidentally, I was already very familiar with oral mucositis, painful ulcers that develop in the mouth and throat, as well as xerostomia (dry mouth). I studied these side effects extensively back in 2006 as part of the due diligence process when I licensed and launched an advanced electrolyte solution called Caphosol® at Cytogen. Available via prescription, Caphosol helped prevent oral mucositis and treat dry mouth. Based on this experience, I knew what to expect from my chemoradiation treatment and planned to incorporate

Caphosol into my arsenal against these debilitating side effects.

During the day, I enrolled in two clinical trials—one for imaging and another for blood tests. The imaging study looked at levels of oxygen deficiency (hypoxia) in the tumor tissue. Hypoxic tumor cells are resistant to radiation and many anticancer drugs, and therefore tumor hypoxia influences the outcome of treatment with radiotherapy, chemotherapy and even surgery. The hope is that ruling out hypoxia in the area of the tumor through imaging could reduce the amount of radiation therapy needed to cure the disease, and thus reduce side effects.

The blood test study could be viewed as a type of "liquid biopsy" designed to detect circulating tumor cells and fragments of tumor DNA that are shed into the blood from the primary tumor and metastatic sites. Analyzing changes in these markers may be able to predict the likelihood of disease recurrence after therapy.

It was a very long day, with my first appointment starting at 9 am and my last one not finishing until around 6 pm. They had whisked me away so quickly at the start of the day that I didn't get to see Lorie much at all. In fact, she got worried that things were taking so long that she asked one of the nurses if she could go back and see me. She was allowed back between my scans, and we had a chance to sit together in a small waiting area for a while. I was very anxious due to all the activity and wearing the radiation mask. Fortunately, Lorie brought my Ativan® (lorazepam) to help calm me down.

Putting aside all of the needle poking and prodding, in addition to my fourth flexible endoscopy procedure, by the end of the day I felt much better knowing the timeframe for starting chemoradiation treatment. It was confirmed for Monday, January 18th, 2016—nearly two months after I first discovered the lump on my neck.

Since I couldn't eat all day due to potential interference with the imaging tests, the best part was grabbing a quick dinner at the Hard Rock Café in Times Square with Lorie before taking the train back to Pennsylvania. We both wanted to be back home, but it would be hours before having a meal if we didn't do it now.

After dinner, during the commute home, Lorie and I held hands and discussed the irony of my situation.

"It's strange, isn't it?" I said with the rattling train wheels clicking rhythmically in the background.

"What's that?"

"I don't know...the fact that I started my professional career with computer programing, then became a broker, analyst, and portfolio manager, and climbed my way to the top as CEO of an oncology-focused biotechnology company—only to be later diagnosed with Stage IV cancer. What are the odds?"

We sat in silence for a minute, reflecting on the situation.

"Honey..." I said, trying to find the right words. "I want you to know that I feel extremely blessed to have you by my side during all this. It sounds cliché, but you're my rock—the one stable thing over the years, especially as my career path twisted and turned. And now, at every doctor's appointment and imaging procedure, you're always right there by my side."

"Just remember your promise," she replied, voice cracking, as the sparkle in her eyes became even more pronounced with newly-formed teardrops.

Long ago, we had envisioned how we would grow old together. Each time we saw a charming, elderly couple holding hands or other public displays of affection, we would both smile warmly and comment how "that will be us." The children would be grown and happily married, while we would be free to travel the world and enjoy each other's company. Lorie had a clear vision for this time, but more importantly how it would end—with her dying first, just like her mother. She didn't want to be the one alone, and so, early in our marriage, she had made me "promise" not to die first. Of course, we both knew that such a decision wasn't ultimately up to me, but to keep her Pollyanna vision for the future intact, I had reluctantly agreed.

We sat quietly the rest of the trip home, our heads resting together.

Chapter Two
Walk with Purpose

———

Around the time my cancer treatment began, I embarked on a journey of self-reflection. It started by pondering my existence and how it might very well be coming to an end in a relatively short period. Not just how it would happen physically—the nauseating, noxious side-effects of the chemoradiation treatment, the inevitable slide of deterioration and increased pain—but the impact on my wife and family, friends, and my fellow-workers.

Frankly, it was pretty lucky that I had even made it into my late 40's. During my teenage years, I had experimented with drugs and alcohol while teaching myself how to play guitar and dreaming of becoming the next David Gilmour or Eddie van Halen. I was also a promiscuous teenager, which in retrospect is likely how I contracted the human papillomavirus that would persist for several decades before causing cancer. Making it through many near-death and reckless experiences during that period now seemed like a minor miracle.

My mind continued wandering back further in time. Isn't that a common phenomenon with people who are facing imminent death? No, I didn't spin back to my first recollections and experiences or re-live highlights, moments of joy, or tragedy. I didn't recall wonderful or terrible stuff that had been long forgotten.

But I did think about how the world I was in today wasn't all that different than when I was born. I'd heard about 1968 from my parents, studied it a little in school, and picked up a lot by osmosis. I knew that the sixties, and especially the year of my birth, had been engraved so powerfully in history. Now, finding myself considering how this year, right now, might be the end for me, I began reading and thinking more about the year of my birth—nearly 50 years ago.

1968 wasn't just the tipping point of the sixties; it was, as Time Inc. called it "the year that changed the world." The decade had started with the inauguration of John F. Kennedy, a young, charismatic, eloquent new president who inspired a tremendous burst of hope and optimism about the possibilities of the future. The civil rights movement, the emergence of black-inspired rock and roll, the Beatles and Rolling Stones—all brought young people together in a counter-culture that challenged the establishment and seemed like it could change things and create an authentic revolution.

But in 1968, the dream of the youth culture began to die. JFK had already been assassinated, and the nation was deeply divided about the Vietnam War. With the failure of Lyndon Johnson and election of Richard Nixon as President, 1968 began to slide into disappointment. Not unlike the present day, the nation seemed to be hurling full speed into chaos and division.

Then two giants of hope, Senator Robert F. Kennedy and Reverend Martin Luther King Jr., were assassinated in 1968, the latter of which resulted in the broadest wave of social unrest since the American Civil War.

In contrast to Martin Luther King Jr.'s non-violent response to injustice in American society, the Black Power Movement came to represent the demand for more immediate violent action to counter American white supremacy. This rising generation of black militant leaders advocated aggressive tactics to counter what they viewed as a profoundly racist and unfair society.

During the period's youth movement, America's middle-class kids became revolutionaries. In April 1968, student rebels stormed the office of president at New York's prestigious Columbia University, forcing the suspension of all classes until New York City police were called and able to restore order. The uprising spread to other campuses across the nation—Princeton, Stony Brook, and Northwestern. Months later, police clashed with young anti-war protesters in Chicago, Illinois, outside the 1968 Democratic National Convention in one of the most severe civil disruptions in U.S. history. Hundreds of protestors were arrested and hundreds more injured.

Another important social crusade was in its early phases in 1968: the feminist movement. Led by activist and author Robin Morgan, women's liberation groups arrived in Atlantic City, New Jersey that year to protest against the Miss America Pageant as exploitative of women in one of the first massive demonstrations of second-wave feminism. Protestors ridiculed the event as a cattle auction, displaying posters of women with their bodies marked up as meat charts with labels such as rib, chuck, round, rump, and loin.

Beyond the ongoing Vietnam War, geopolitical tensions escalated in the Asia Regions in January 1968 when North Korea seized the U.S.S. *Pueblo*, a U.S. spy ship, and held its 82 sailors as hostages. During the 11-month ordeal, members of the vessel were jailed, tortured, and starved before their release on December 23, 1968.

Sadly, five decades later many of the issues making headlines remain the same. As philosopher George Santayana once said, "Those who cannot learn from history are doomed to repeat it." However, it makes me sad to think that this reflects a failure of the social movements from the late 1960's.

Protestors and rioters spoke loudly at the time, but perhaps they weren't heard. I can still hear echoes of their voices in today's world, where racial tensions, police brutality, youth counterculture, gender equality, and geopolitical tensions persist.

While we are a long way from 1968, there has been scant progress over nearly five decades towards becoming a Utopian society where people live together in harmony with universal values and customs.

OK. That was the world when I was born in 1968, but I also thought about where I'd come from, the family who had created me, beginning with my parents. In particular, I considered how they equipped me for an unusual journey from teenage hell-raiser to a computer programmer, investment advisor, husband, father, CEO of an oncology-focused biotechnology company, and finally—a terminal cancer patient facing his mortality.

In 1966, during his senior year of college at DePauw University in Greencastle, Indiana, my father, George "Ted" Becker, first met and dated my mother, JoAnn Chinn. They met at the investment firm Wayne Hummer & Co. He worked there during summer break from school, and she worked as a keypunch operator. They got married in 1967, within a year of my father's graduation from college.

My father's father, George Roth Becker, was the first of three Becker generations to work at Wayne Hummer & Co. and enjoyed a very successful 43-year business career there. Thanks to a family relationship with Mr. Wayne Hummer that began in his boyhood, my grandfather George joined the firm in 1936. There are rumors that he was a bit of a hell-raiser and that his parents paid his salary at Wayne Hummer to keep him working and out of trouble.

George became the office manager in 1948, general partner in 1954, then rose to managing partner and remained in that position until his retirement in 1979. He was a very hard worker and seldom made it home on the weekends. My father, Ted, would bring him change of clothes on Saturdays and eventually was offered a job in the mailroom when he turned 16, marking the start of his 36-year career with the firm.

Mr. Hummer was president of LaSalle National Bank, and his close friend and the bank's trust officer, George Barnes, would occasionally discuss a problem facing most small banks in those days—the issue of ethics in the bond brokerage industry.

The problem arose because representatives from Chicago and New York investment companies would call on the small-town banks to sell securities. These salesmen didn't act only as a broker agent when giving investment advice and executing orders for the banks, but would often be involved in the actual underwriting of the securities they were selling. Therefore, there was the potential for a conflict of interest.

During the 1920's numerous small-town banks and individuals relied on advice from these investment company representatives. The result was that many of these investors made unwise, and sometimes disastrous, decisions when buying securities from these companies.

Mr. Hummer avoided the problem by refusing to deal with these salesmen. He bought bonds on his own and even began to help other bankers make wise choices. However, the ethics of the bond salesmen bothered him, and the conversations with Mr. Barnes began to nurture a dream of someday starting a brokerage firm to give small-town bankers a more ethical standard of service. The appeal in doing so was the opportunity to right a wrong. That motivation was an essential part of the story, for it illustrates the fact that altruistic motives drive some entrepreneurs.

It took courage, determination, and foresight to open a new investment firm in 1931, but that's precisely what Hummer and Barnes did. Over the years, the firm came to represent the highest standards of ethics and integrity combined with an uncommon level of personal service and attention.

During his tenure at Wayne Hummer & Co., my grandfather found a way to simplify trading with New York exchanges from Wayne Hummer's offices in Chicago. He was among the early proponents for computerized accounting at the Midwest Stock Exchange, the precursor to the Chicago Stock Exchange, where he served as chairman.

In addition to his work at Wayne Hummer, he served as village president of Glen Ellyn, an affluent suburban village in DuPage County, Illinois. He also served as chairman of DuPage Bank & Trust Company, president of the Glen Oak Country Club, and as scoutmaster of Troop 44 in Glen Ellyn. He was also an excellent and highly competitive golfer, although I can't for the life of me figure out when he was able to make time for it. He died on Halloween in 2000 from pneumonia and complications from Alzheimer's disease at the age of 84.

Knowing that he could be drafted due to the ongoing Vietnam War, my father enlisted for Officer Candidate School (Quartermaster) and was commissioned a 2nd lieutenant approximately a year later. After completing Army schooling, he was stationed in Fort Riley, Kansas during his several years of service. My parents lived there in a Post Supply building that was converted into apartments.

For the next five months, JoAnn somehow dismissed nausea and modest weight gain. It wasn't until a subsequent doctor's visit that she learned, much to her surprise, that she was pregnant. I was born November 12th, 1968 at the Irwin Army Hospital—a month before the first manned mission to the moon.

After completion of his military obligations in 1969, we returned to the suburbs of Chicago. My father resumed working full-time at Wayne Hummer in the internal audit and control department. It was apparent even at an early age that my parents had clearly defined roles and responsibilities. Dad was to be the breadwinner while my mother's job was to stay at home and raise the children. Not an unusual arrangement for the time and, in truth, it worked quite well. My mom was warm, sensitive, and most likely to say "yes," in contrast to my father, who was the opposite. It was Dad who dished out punishment, while Mom was the consummate peacemaker. Despite their different personalities and parenting techniques, I never questioned whether or not they loved me, albeit each in their way, and I had a generally healthy and happy childhood.

In June 1973, my sister Brandy was born. I would love to say that I welcomed her into the world with open arms, but that would be a lie. An otherwise healthy infant, she was a colicky baby who would cry for hours—often in the evening. Not only that, I quickly discovered that I was no longer an only child receiving 100 percent of my parent's attention. Not even close. Our relationship may have got off to a rough start, but I always loved her. We grew closer once she let us all sleep through the night.

My world changed at the age of twelve when my parents convened a rare family meeting.

"Children," my mother began. "We have some sad news for you."

Brandy and I sat in silence, wondering what was coming next.

"Your father and I," Mom went on, "are getting a divorce."

I was numb. All sorts of crazy thoughts raced through my head. Did we do something wrong? Would my sister and I be orphans now? Would we have to move, change schools, and lose all of our friends?

Finally, I was able to speak.

"What's going to happen to us? Where will we live?"

"Your mother is going to stay in the house," Dad said, "and I'm getting an apartment in Chicago, near the office."

I didn't know what to say. It seemed like a bad dream. My parents were complete opposites, and to this day it is hard to imagine the chemistry that somehow united them in the first place, but it had seemed to work. How could they end their marriage?

"We've discussed the matter," my dad continued, "and feel that it makes the most sense for you and your sister to live at home here with your mother and visit me on a regular schedule at my new place in Chicago."

"You can stay overnight at his apartment on weekends and some of the holidays," my mother added, trying to soften the blow.

And that was it. Until that point in time, I had a typical middle-class childhood. Now, my family began a new and much more difficult life together.

Following the divorce, one silver lining was that Brandy and I quickly learned to depend on each other. We developed a typical brother/sister relationship, meaning that we alternated between being best friends and greatest enemies throughout a constant power struggle to get the most attention.

When we joined forces and were each other's partner in crime, we brought out the worst in each other. In fact, our Halloween and April Fool's Day pranks on my mother were legendary—much to her chagrin. Other victims of our antics included our maternal grandparents, Ronald and Eileen Chinn, who lived in a condominium in Buffalo Grove, Illinois. Growing up, Brandy and I spent a fair amount of time fishing on their lake during the summer and swimming in their indoor pool in the winter. They were avid golfers, so we convinced them to take us to see the new golf movie *Caddyshack* that was released that year. I'll never forget the embarrassed look on their faces as they hurried the two of us down the aisle to exit the theater as the reason for the movie's "restricted" rating came bouncing across the screen in all their glory. They didn't let us pick out which movie to see ever again.

———

I remembered something else that happened later the same year, 1980, when I was still twelve years old. It was winter, and my father had just moved into a condominium after the divorce. The building was located in Printer's Row, an up-and-coming neighborhood south of the Chicago downtown area known as The Loop. The proximity to Wayne Hummer meant my dad could walk to work each day rather than commuting on the train from the Northwest suburbs where we once lived happily together as a family.

That year, my sister and I spent Christmas Eve with him at his condo and then we returned home the following day to celebrate Christmas with our mother. The holiday was a special time for her. She loved baking Christmas cookies, homemade fudge, powdered snowball cookies, gingerbread men, and much more. We often joked that she should be called JoAnn "Baker" instead of Becker.

On Christmas Eve, after dining together in the small kitchen area of Dad's condo, we gathered to open presents in the living room. From under the tree, I grabbed the largest gift addressed to me and began frantically unwrapping the festive Christmas paper and tugging on the red ribbon until it snapped. My eyes grew wide as I realized with glee that the gift from my father was a Radio Shack Tandy TRS-80 Color Computer.

I slid the slick, silver unit with a built-in keyboard from its box, removed the protective white Styrofoam packing, and began connecting the various cables. The Color Computer didn't come with a built-in floppy disk drive or even a video monitor. In fact, it's hard to believe that the Color Computer was designed to save and load programs and data from a standard audio cassette deck. It had radio frequency (RF) converters that could be connected to the antenna inputs of a television with a simple screwdriver. The computer signal was received on channel 3 or 4, so I turned the dial on my father's television accordingly and was mesmerized as a single blinking cursor appeared in the upper left corner of the blank, neon green screen.

With all of the gifts unwrapped and resulting mess cleaned up, my sister and father retired for the evening. The condo was dark except for the soft glow from the television screen and tungsten city lights below, which seemed to extend forever through the large windows.

It was my chance to stay up and begin learning "Tandy Color BASIC," which is what the machine used as its programming language instead of the more popular Microsoft BASIC. In a short time, I was able to program the computer to perform simple tasks and play games. It was my first serious foray into computer programming, one of several self-taught skills that would serve me well in subsequent years.

I was interested in science and technology from an early age, but my passion for computers had grown exponentially. I spent hours playing favorite games such as Pong, Adventure, and Space Invaders, and also hanging out at video arcades with my friends. Now I had a personal computer that I could program to do anything.

Delusions of grandeur swirled in my adolescent mind as I envisioned myself starring in an American Cold War science-fiction film where I would find a back door into a central military computer and nearly start World War III. Those fantasies came to an abrupt ending, however, when I realized that with a standard memory configuration consisting of four kilobytes of RAM, my dad's coffee maker had a better chance of starting a global thermonuclear war than my new computer. Too bad for me, world domination would have to wait.

Even with the financial support she received from Dad, money was tight after the divorce. Not having worked for more than fifteen years, Mom took a part-time job sorting plastic pieces coming off an assembly belt around the holidays to earn some extra money. Only after ensuring that my sister and I had a hot meal for dinner, she'd leave for a few hours and be back home around bedtime, often with red and blistered fingers from handling the hot pieces of freshly molded plastic.

That Christmas day, much to our joy and surprise, my sister and I each got black and white television sets for our bedrooms. It turned out that she had suffered through that terrible job to provide us with holiday presents; something we would never forget. Putting others before herself was normal for Mom, especially when it came to her children.

There's a lot more that I remember about the year 1980. The high-resolution images of Saturn from NASA's space probe *Voyager I*, the eruption of Mount St. Helens, Led Zeppelin breaking up due to the death of their drummer John Bonham, and Ronald Reagan being elected as president. Most vividly, however, I remember crying in my bedroom on December 8th after learning on the radio that John Lennon had been shot dead outside his apartment in New York City.

What I didn't know at the time was that across the country in Princeton, New Jersey, venture capitalist Robert F. Johnston was busy founding Cytogen Corporation, one of the first biotechnology companies focusing on the emerging field of monoclonal antibodies that was stirring widespread interest within the scientific community in the 1980s. Monoclonal antibodies, or mAbs, are biological agents that can bind to specific proteins on cancer cells and other targets in the body.

Robert recruited Dr. Thomas McKearn from the University of Pennsylvania, who had just written a book on monoclonal antibodies. He developed methods to link mAbs to solid surfaces for diagnostic tests for sexually transmitted diseases and blood separation processes, to radioisotopes for imaging and therapy, and to chemotherapies for cancer treatment. Robert also brought in Steve Chubb as Cytogen's first CEO.

Cytogen's work on monoclonal antibodies to kill tumors was considered cutting-edge research at that time. Who would have guessed that 21 years later, I would become CEO of Cytogen?

————

Shortly after my parents' divorce, I entered my teenage years with reckless abandon and became a challenging child for my mother to raise. Too much for any two parents to handle, let alone a single mother trying to earn a living while raising two young kids.

I moved out of the house and was soon living in a small studio apartment over a used automobile dealership in Arlington Heights, Illinois. I dropped out of William Fremd High School one year before graduating so that I could work full-time supporting myself, taking a relatively mindless job doing microfilm scanning and paper document conversion services at a local firm. It paid the rent and helped my recreational habits. The company also didn't mind my shoulder-length hair and earrings or have a strict dress code. Wearing jeans to work was acceptable; life was good.

Approaching my twenties, however, I realized the need to straighten up and start building a future for myself. Instead of being among Fremd's graduating class of 1987, I obtained my General Educational Development (GED) the following year. Jumping into a career without first securing a college degree was the best thing that ever happened to me and other talented self-starters, including entrepreneurs, artists, and even a former U.S. surgeons general. It's not for everyone, however, and I'm a firm believer in the benefit of a good education.

In 1988, I reached out nervously to my father about potential employment at Wayne Hummer. We always had a somewhat strained relationship, and the divorce didn't make things easier. But he was very conscientious about keeping the lines of communication open in both good times and bad. I always knew he loved me; he told me so and showed it in his ways. But we never shared any real deep conversations or personal feelings.

For example, he didn't tell me what kinds of problems he wrestled with, what he felt, or what it meant to him to be a good man, husband, or father. All my life I've felt like I had to make it up for myself, and I've never been sure I got it quite right.

One thing is for sure; Dad instilled his strong work ethics in me, and he got them from his father. George Roth Becker was known for barking phrases at his four sons like "quit your loafing." He once told my dad that "if it ever comes down to promoting you or someone else and both were equal, I'd promote the other guy."

Entitlement and nepotism were four-letter words in the Becker family. Everything was to be earned—and nothing came easy. In retrospect, I wish that I adopted a bit more of this parenting style later in life with my children.

Not surprisingly, I would be put through the full interview process at Wayne Hummer—there would be no free ride for a Becker. In preparation, I shed a tear as a barber transformed my shoulder-length mane into a short, combed-back haircut suitable for a professional career. Then Dad took me shopping for business attire, and I walked away with several pairs of tailored dress pants, shirts, dress shoes, and ties.

The interview process at Wayne Hummer was terrifying. To avoid any signs of favoritism, my father didn't participate at all. In fact, the human resource coordinator greeted me in the reception area when I arrived and escorted me directly to a small room to fill out paperwork. She also administered a typing test to gauge speed and accuracy, which my father had forewarned was a requirement for employment in the computer department. Fortunately, between playing with computers and taking required typing classes during high school, I was pretty fast and accurate.

On April 14th, 1988, nearly a decade after my grandfather George's retirement, I became the third-generation Becker to work at Wayne Hummer. I was offered a starting position working in the computer department under the tutelage of Paul Carroll, who headed the unit. His older brother, Douglas Carroll, was also employed at Wayne Hummer where he worked closely with his father, John D. Carroll, in sales. Both brothers were quite interested in computer programming, so Douglas spent considerable time in the office that Paul and I shared with another department. It was entertaining to watch them frequently spar over who's coding approach was fastest or most efficient.

Similar to my grandfather's background, John Carroll came to Wayne Hummer through his relationship with one of the firm's founders, George Barnes. John became a successful partner and later brought Douglas and Paul into the company.

———

Early one morning, with few employees having arrived yet, I passed Dad during my daily walk around the office distributing portfolio reports to the brokers. He stopped momentarily and took me aside.

"Michael," he said in a stern but hushed voice so only I could hear him.

"Yes, Dad?" I replied.

"Walk with purpose."

"What?" I said, now puzzled.

"If you meander from point A to point B," he explained, "you might give people the incorrect impression that you're lazy or bored."

Judging by the blank expression on my face, he could tell I still wasn't getting his point, so he elaborated.

"If you walk briskly and with intent, as though you were running late for an important meeting, you'll give others the impression that you have confidence and importance."

"So..." I began.

"So, walk with purpose!" he said and turned on his heel to continue what he was doing.

I didn't know it at the time, but it was a defining moment for me. The simple notion that one's actions, expressions, or appearance could influence perception by others—either positively or negatively—was quite astute and ultimately useful. And while perhaps resented at the time, I came to appreciate later in life just how vital his constant pushing to "do better," and the lack of entitlement helped me achieve my eventual success in life. Perhaps it's why my grandparents' four sons were each highly successful as well.

Meanwhile, programming work was well underway by the time I joined the firm. Douglas and Paul collaborated on creating a front office sales automation (FOSA) computer program for Wayne Hummer with the added hope that it could eventually be sold or licensed to other brokerage firms. As a broker himself, Douglas had unique insight to help shape the FOSA program to service the firm's needs.

Paul gave me various small programming projects related to FOSA and helped to develop my technical knowledge. The time I spent learning and working with the two brothers significantly improved my computer skills, with the consequence of making me much more marketable to other local brokerage firms. It was a very conscious and unselfish decision by Paul, as he always viewed my time at Wayne Hummer as a stepping stone and not a destination.

In just over a year working at Wayne Hummer, I received an unsolicited telephone call from a recruiter who was representing prominent New York-based investment bank Kidder, Peabody & Co. The firm was looking to fill the newly created position of manager of information systems for their Chicago branch. While I wasn't actively seeking to leave Wayne Hummer, the job at Kidder represented a promotion in both title and pay, which I couldn't afford to turn down. I would be in charge of establishing the computer department and applying the programming skills learned at Wayne Hummer to automate various front office functions.

Leaving the "family business" was a tough decision, but the allure of starting my computer fiefdom was far too great to resist. Besides, Wayne Hummer was a relatively small player in the brokerage world, and I knew they would have difficulty competing with larger firms like Kidder for talent, compensation, and growth opportunities.

I arrived at a decision completely on my own. The next morning, *having not yet mastered how to walk with purpose*, I sauntered apprehensively down the long corridor to my father's office. No matter when I came there, he always appeared busy—concentrating on documents, talking on the phone, or tapping away frantically on the keys of his adding machine.

In typical fashion, the conversation was quite short and to the point. Dad didn't exhibit any emotion at the news of my imminent departure from the firm that carried a long tradition of Becker's, starting with my grandfather. The lack of reaction or extensive discussion gave me the distinct impression that he didn't care whether or not I worked at the firm. Or worse, that he was angry with me over the decision to leave. Only much, much later in life would I gain insight into his thought process at the time.

"I know that I always wanted you to be happy in any path you chose...and was fortunate that I was able to give you an opportunity to have a job and get work experience," he informed me later. "I was proud to have my son working at the firm which carried on a long tradition of Becker's, but you were and are an intelligent, quick-witted, independent thinker, and I knew you would succeed at whatever you decided to do. I believe what *challenges* you motivates and drives you. I had absolutely no hard feelings, not disappointed, nor angry...and was happy that you were succeeding and being recognized for your talents and capabilities."

The conversation with Paul Carroll was more representative of what I expected from the situation. Returning to our shared office after meeting with Dad, Paul could tell from the expression on my face that something was up. I wear my heart on my sleeve.

"Paul, I received an unsolicited offer from Kidder, Peabody to head up their budding computer department here in Chicago and will be resigning from Wayne Hummer."

"I see," he replied.

"I'm giving two weeks notice so that the transition goes smoothly. I should be able to wrap-up any outstanding projects within that period."

"We'll try to get along without you," he said jokingly, attempting to diffuse the tension. Sure, the new job offer was proof that Paul had succeeded in mentoring me. But I knew he still must be somewhat disappointed to see me go.

There was a sense of comradery among Paul, Douglas, and me. We were each the progeny of partners at the firm and lived in the shadows of our successful fathers. Additionally, we were all somewhat the black sheep of our families; quirky and nerdy because of our deep interest in computers and software.

Working in sales, Paul's older brother Douglas was slightly different. He was better able to adapt to his surroundings like a chameleon. More importantly, he was tenacious and mastered anything that interested or challenged him—which would eventually include hobbies such as photography and scuba diving in addition to becoming a very successful stockbroker. After being hired by his father in 1976, he rose to the position of partner within a decade.

During the time he spent with us talking about technology in the computer department, his presence was that of a peer. He would converse about the latest and greatest gadgets or computer hardware with great enthusiasm and passion. He possessed *confidence*, some might argue arrogance, which also allowed him to excel as a stockbroker. Sureness was something I didn't have at the time. But I related to his mastery of all subjects that interested him, especially whenever he was thrown into the deep end of a pool, and I felt we had this in common.

———

I started working at Kidder, Peabody & Co. in the summer of 1989 and quickly earned the trust and respect of Steven Satkamp, managing director and head of the Chicago branch. A few years' prior, the firm had installed a market-data system nationally that used proprietary dumb terminals and software to support the firm's stockbrokers. Some of the brokers in Chicago were unhappy with the limitations of the system, however, and I give Steven a lot of credit for recognizing and addressing this situation.

With Steven's support, I was able to secure state-of-the-art computer equipment and software to build a working financial reporting system that exclusively served the Chicago branch office. Unfortunately, the computer department at the firm's New York headquarters was racing to introduce a competing solution that would be rolled out nationally. Since the Chicago branch was also a beta testing site for New York's system, Steven arranged a meeting between the competing group and me to learn about their project, present my application, and try to convince them why capturing and storing financial data offered a potentially better solution.

Having just turned 21, I was young, naïve, and had never even traveled alone. Although I had recently moved to a studio apartment on Lake Shore Drive in Chicago from the suburbs to be closer to work, New York seemed much more substantial, faster and foreboding. Kidder arranged for me to stay at the prestigious Downtown Athletic Club, a private social and athletic club located less than half a mile south of the World Trade Center.

I arrived on a Sunday, which gave me a brief amount of time to play tourist. But New York's financial district was a proverbial ghost town on the weekends. I didn't know enough about Manhattan to make my way towards Greenwich Village and Midtown for more action. Besides, it was the middle of winter and there was light snow on the ground.

Nonetheless, I ended up purchasing a disposable film camera and took a tour of the Statue of Liberty. After climbing my way to the top, staring at the vastness of Gotham below me on that dreary winter day, I never felt so alone, so, small, so cold.

The next morning, a car service arrived at the hotel and took me the offices of Kidder, Peabody & Co. My meeting was with Calvin Emory, manager of information technology, and Mary Uslander, assistant vice president and manager of retail technology. We had spoken previously on the phone, but this was our first personal interaction.

It had snowed again during the night, and the curbs were a slushy, wet mess. It made me regret even further my poor clothing selection for the trip. While I had several better options available, in a stroke of youthful brilliance, I had decided to pack my best *"Miami Vice"* jacket and pants in one of the show's approved colors: bright blue. With a coordinated salmon-colored shirt, I must have been quite a sight in the middle of winter. Worse yet, the cold, wet snow easily penetrated my black moccasins as I stepped out of the car upon arrival at Kidder, Peabody's office.

As we exchanged pleasantries, I noticed that Calvin appeared to be in his forties, but his hairline gave the impression that he was a bit older. He was tall with a medium frame. His movements were supple, graceful, and athletic. His conversation tended to be sprinkled with novelty and wit. As a result, he came across as a consummate salesman. But beneath the quick tongue and charisma, I thought he was a bit of a dilettante. While he had sold Kidder, Peabody & Co. on the attractiveness of his group's product offering, I was concerned that some important details hadn't yet been addressed. We sparred for a while as I made a case for the software system that I had created.

"Regarding functionality, the brokers in our branch feel that the ability to retrieve historical prices, allowing them to recreate the value of a client's portfolio as of a particular date, is critical," I argued, "especially for estate valuations."

Instead of engaging in a discussion of the facts, however, Calvin turned on the magic with a gleam in his eye, "You *know* something, Michael, you'd be a *great* addition to our team here in New York. As we roll our system out nationally, we're going to need more resources. A young, good-looking guy like you, living in the Big Apple; *think* about the possibilities."

I was youthful, but not stupid. I figured Calvin was trying to lure me away from the Chicago office as a way to eliminate a potential thorn in his side. However, Calvin had found a creative solution to his problem (me) and moved swiftly to advance his agenda. Without notice, he pressed the speed-dial button on his speakerphone and called my boss in Chicago.

"Hello, this is Calvin Emory from New York. May I please speak with Steven?" he said to the assistant answering the line.

"Sure, just a moment," she replied.

"Hello, Calvin. I trust you're treating our guest well?" said the familiar voice on the other end.

"But of *course*," Calvin replied, trying to sound genuine. "We've been having some *excellent* discussions. Thank you so much for arranging this meeting. In fact, we wanted to run an idea by you. What do you think about Michael transferring to New York to help us roll out the new system? It seems a shame to limit his talents to Chicago."

"Boy, I don't know, Calvin," Steven replied, "we've got some high-producing brokers here that rely heavily upon the reports that only Michael's system can produce right now. I was hoping that you could find a way to work together and perhaps incorporate some of his capabilities into your new system. But Michael has a say in all of this, so continue your discussions. He can debrief me upon his return."

Unfortunately, Steven had inadvertently left a crack in door and Calvin used the remainder of our time together to feed my ego and talk up New York. Knowing that if he could entice me with the big lights and bright city, I would return to

Steven favorably inclined, or perhaps even beg, to make the transfer.

I felt defeated. The Big, Bad Apple had beaten me. A short while after my return to Chicago, in their haste to try and extinguish the need for both me and my program, New York's new system was formally rolled out. It was a botched launch with significant bugs and feature limitations. The Chicago branch office's largest commission producers revolted. Steven supported allowing my software to run in parallel for anyone that wanted to continue using it until the "new" system could match its capabilities, which ultimately would take several years.

Attempting to scratch an itch I had since first seeing Oliver Stone's movie *Wall Street* back in 1987, I approached Steven about becoming a stockbroker.

"I'm sorry Michael," he explained in a polite but firm manner, "but the firm normally only hires Ivy League graduates with extensive, affluent connections."

To be fair, I wasn't a good fit for the firm at the time, but that didn't lessen the blow to my ego. It did make me want to become a broker even more, however. Telling me that I couldn't do something was a sure-fire way to motivate me to succeed and overcome obstacles.

Steven did throw me a bone by allowing me to take the requisite Registered Representative (Series 7) exam, which required sponsorship from a firm like Kidder, Peabody & Co. I was provided home-study materials and passed the test in May 1990. As a result, I was allowed to buy and sell stocks strictly for my account, which only fueled my appetite to become a broker. Not having much investible money at the time, I dabbled in risky casino and pharmaceutical stocks that traded on the Pink Sheets. Typically, companies are on the Pink Sheets because either they are too small to be listed on a national exchange or they don't want to make their budgets and accounting statements public. Unfortunately, such companies are usually penny stocks and are often targets of price manipulation. With stellar investments such as DynaGen, Inc. and Nona Morelli's II, Inc., I never made a dime and put my Wall Street career on the backburner.

My vast technology empire soon doubled with the hiring of a longtime childhood friend, Steve Harmon. The firm knew that I needed some additional help and allowed me to hire him based on my recommendation. I'd known Steve since we were both at Paddock Elementary School in Palatine, Illinois. Like me, he was good with computers and I mentored him in programming—just like Paul and Douglas had done for me at Wayne Hummer. To ease his commute, Steve ended up being my roommate in Chicago during the weekdays. He brought his old Commodore 64 computer and after work each day we drank and played vintage video games; it was a fun time.

Steve had a steady girlfriend at the time, so he'd commute back to the suburbs on weekends to spend time with her. Having grown quite tired of the bar dating scene in Chicago, I asked Steve to inquire if she had any available friends, hoping maybe I could wrangle a date.

Chapter Three
Just One Night

———

Quite by coincidence, the mother of Steve's girlfriend was a teacher at Paddock Elementary School. Steve informed me that she offered to make an introduction to a colleague, Lorie Statland, a young single woman who taught kindergarten there.

I kept pestering Steve to see if Lorie was interested in going on a blind date with me. After several inquiries, he reluctantly informed me that Lorie wasn't interested. Most people would give up at this point, but not me.

"Tell her it's only one night of her life," I finally said to Steve in a last-ditch effort. "If she doesn't have a good time, we never have to see each other again."

Apparently "it's only one night" was persuasive and Steve provided me with Lorie's phone number. Given her past reluctance, I was quite nervous about phoning her.

One evening, after getting up enough nerve, I pressed the telephone to my ear as I dialed the number Steve had given me.

Three, four, five, six rings. Finally, someone picked up the phone.

"Hello..." the woman answered, sounding a bit breathless.

"Hello, umm, may I please speak with Lorie?"

"Yes, this is she."

She sounded frantic and definitely out of breath.

"It's Michael Becker. Steve gave me your number, and I was calling to set up our—"

"Can I call you right back?" she interrupted. "My rabbit just got behind the entertainment center and I have to get him out!"

"Rabbit?"

"Yes, my pet bunny, P.J." she exclaimed, still out of breath. "I'll have to call you back..."

She hung up abruptly.

I stared at the phone in disbelief, having no choice but to wait and see. Maybe Lorie would never call back. Maybe she'd changed her mind about going out on a blind date. Or worse, perhaps one of my former teachers still worked at

Paddock Elementary and remembered me as a troublemaker. Maybe I was nervous and a little nuts.

Lorie called back in just a few minutes and on August 14th, 1990 we had our marathon first date. Living in downtown Chicago at the time, I had little need for a car, so Lorie had agreed to drive into the city. I suggested that we meet at my apartment building, in part to dazzle her with my prestigious Lake Shore Drive location, but also since there were plenty of restaurants and bars within a short radius.

When the front desk phoned to announce that a guest had arrived, I took the back stairwell instead of the main elevator and placed a dozen red roses on one of the chairs in the lobby before approaching Lorie from behind. During our initial phone call, she had informed me that our date fell upon her "half birthday." Not familiar with the concept, she explained to me that every child with a summer birthday (when school isn't in session) gets a classroom celebration for their half-birthdays at most preschools and elementary schools. It only seemed appropriate to give her flowers. On the accompanying card, I simply wrote, "Happy ½ birthday and to new beginnings...Michael"

I was thrilled when I saw her the first time. Lorie was thin and beautiful with dark brown hair and big, round brown eyes that twinkled every time she smiled or laughed. I vowed at that very moment to make it my life's goal to cause her to smile as often as I could, so that I could see them sparkle.

Importantly, she was entirely different from the other women I had dated in recent years. She had an established career and came across as intelligent, secure, and independent, which I found very attractive. She was also perky and laughed at all my bad jokes.

I was smitten.

As we exited the lobby, I pointed to the flowers resting on the chair.

"Look, someone must have left these here for you."

We started with cocktails at Dos Hermanos in the Sears Tower before dining at Houston's, an upscale restaurant on Rush Street, just off the city's Magnificent Mile. It was a gorgeous summer evening, so after drinks and dinner, we took a horse-drawn carriage ride near the Water Tower on Michigan Avenue.

At the end of the night, we walked back to my apartment building with a doggie bag from dinner. Since Lorie loves animals, we stopped briefly upstairs so she could meet Missy, a German Shepherd mix that I had recently rescued from the Anti-Cruelty Society in Chicago.

It turned out to be much more than "just one night." We ended up dating and falling in love, with the only bumps in the road emanating from some of our differences. Lorie is just over two years older than me and Jewish, which I wasn't when we met, nor did I have a car or a college degree at the time. And while I had since outgrown it, my previous "bad boy" persona was a stark contrast to Lorie, whose worst sin in life was angrily pulling her mother's flowers from the yard once when she was a little girl. Against this backdrop, I had the Herculean task of continually proving to her father, Jack Statland, that I was a good match for his beautiful daughter.

"Of course, I would have preferred that you were a nice, young Jewish attorney," Jack stated matter-of-factly during one of our very early interactions in the kitchen of his home in Skokie.

Worldly and well educated, Jack was a man noted (*feared*) for his traditionally male interests and activities. You never wondered what was on his mind, as he spoke bluntly and with unabashed honesty. He had served his country, enjoyed watching contact sports such as football, loved a good cigar, and was passionate about automobiles—especially his bright red, restored 1968 Pontiac Firebird convertible. He was also widely regarded, as Rabbi Victor Weissberg would later recall at his funeral, as "a lover of love."

Lorie's mother, Rose Statland, sadly passed away due to complications arising from heart surgery in her 50's. I never had the pleasure of meeting Rose, but from everything I have seen and heard, Lorie is the spitting image of her.

Being with Lorie made me want to be a smarter, better, and more educated person, and I knew that my lack of college degree bothered her. Neither one of us enjoyed our early years in school, which had inspired Lorie to become a schoolteacher in the first place. She knew firsthand how much of an impact a teacher could make on a young student—determining whether or not they stay in school, shaping their self-esteem, helping them discover subjects that are of interest.

Quitting my job to return to school wasn't an option, so I enrolled at DePaul University's School for New Learning in early 1991. Through evening classes, the college offered undergraduate and graduate programs designed to meet the needs of working adults.

Six months after our first date, on February 2nd, 1991, I got down on one knee during another carriage ride in downtown Chicago and asked her to marry me. Happily, she said yes. Afterwards we went to the John Hancock Observatory for a scenic view of the city. Lorie used a pay phone to call her family and share the good news.

Being a confirmed Lutheran, but not overly religious, I took note of one of Jack's many unsolicited opinions that same-faith marriages are "just easier," and decided to convert to Judaism in advance of having a traditional Jewish wedding. We attended the requisite educational sessions during the conversion process. With a ceremonial drop of blood and subsequent full immersion into a mikvah pool containing 200 gallons of what was, in my perception, not very clean kosher rainwater, I officially became a Member of the Tribe.

We were married under a chuppah and broke the traditional glass in an unpretentious wedding at the Orrington

Hotel in Evanston, Illinois in the spring of 1992. Looking back, I was especially blessed to have all sets of grandparents able to attend the event.

Lorie's father graciously gave us a lump sum of money as a wedding gift, which he said we could allocate as desired to pay for the wedding or more practical purchases, such as a down payment on a home. So, we had a simple wedding, lovely honeymoon in Hawaii, and had enough left over for a down payment on a tiny, one-story house at the end of a cul-de-sac in Evanston that summer.

Our house was small, but it had character. The prior owners recently renovated the interior in an art deco style that appealed to both of us. In contrast to the inside, there was a spacious backyard where our dog, Missy, could play.

The location was a quick commute to her father's house in Skokie, Illinois and close to the train for my daily commute to work in Chicago. We could only afford one car at the time, so Lorie would drop me off at the Evanston train station in the morning before heading to Palatine to teach. In the evening, she would pick me up at the station and we'd head back home for dinner.

————

I was making a reasonably good living doing computer programming, but I felt that I could earn more money in the long-term by becoming a stockbroker. I asked Lorie to set aside some time for a discussion one evening, which would become the first in a series of conversations during our decades of marriage known as "The Talks."

"Honey, you know I've always been interested in becoming a stockbroker," I started the conversation. "I firmly believe that in the long run, there's more financial upside for us in that career path. However, I've done some research, and unfortunately, there would be some short-term pain as I work to establish myself."

"Just how much pain are we talking about?" she replied with a hefty dose of skepticism.

"There's a local brokerage office that pays minimum wage throughout the training phase, which appears to last about six months. After that, I'll get a modest draw against future commissions for a short period, but it depends on how quickly I can grow my client base, as all of the earnings are based on sales. I think I can get back to earning what I make now and potentially more within a year or so."

"Hmm...that's a long time," she said, still digesting the proposition. "What about Wayne Hummer? Could you get a better offer there?"

"I discussed it at length with my dad, but the firm isn't a good fit for new brokers without an established base of clients. Besides, there is something to be said for doing this on my own."

Since inception, Wayne Hummer had a firm policy against active solicitation of business. Instead, it offered many special services to attract customers, such as its free market letters (Bank Bond Comment Letter and the Stock Market Comment Letter). The firm also offered toll-free numbers to present and potential customers, provided portfolio evaluation and analysis, and handled, without charge, estate valuations and transfers of securities for lawyers and bankers located in smaller communities.

"OK," Lorie said. "I guess if I got a part-time job in addition to teaching full-time, we could make it work. I know this is something you've been interested in for quite some time. Besides, I think you'd be good at sales."

"But you're already teaching religious school Sunday mornings?"

"That still leaves Saturdays and evenings," she shrugged with that twinkle in her eye and a warm smile on her face. She knew that being a stockbroker was what I wanted at the time and she'd do whatever it took to help make it happen. It eventually included her also doing bookkeeping on Saturday mornings for her dad's trucking business, Jack Statland Express, to bring in extra money.

With her support, I applied at the Chicago branch of Gruntal & Co., a boutique investment banking and brokerage firm based in New York City. Before its acquisition in 2002, the firm was among the oldest independent investment banking houses in the U.S. They were also one of the few local firms willing to "train" an individual to become a telemarketer...err...stockbroker. Much to his amusement, Lorie's dad wouldn't say the firm's name without dramatically emphasizing the "Grrrr" and sounding as though he was severely constipated. He did it in jest, and it made us chuckle every time.

In the summer of 1993, I started my apprenticeship at Gruntal & Co. under the joint tutelage of two young brokers. In contrast to the decent salary I was making as a computer programmer, Gruntal paid me $4.25 per hour (minimum wage) during the time that I received my training and took the necessary regulatory exams, which lasted around six months.

I started out as a "dialer," which as the name implies, meant my job was to dial the phone using a list of prospects. If the prospect answered the phone directly, or I was successful in getting past a gatekeeper, I simply said "please hold" before passing the call to one of my two mentors. They would then "qualify" the prospect and determine whether or not they invested in the stock market and would be potentially interested in hearing investment ideas from us in the near future.

Finally, after having mastered the art of dialing and qualifying, I would be faced with the arduous task of opening a certain number of new client accounts within a six-month timeframe. As soon as each new account was opened and the transaction payment cleared, the client would be distributed alternately between the two established brokers who mentored me as the firm's repayment for their investment of time and effort in training me. Upon completion of this final task, I would then be released on my own as a stockbroker—starting from scratch to prospect on my own again. With no book of clients. In a commission pay environment.

Throughout my six-month training process, I averaged making around 300 telephone calls per day. After accounting for busy signals, hang-ups, and other roadblocks, it took that many calls to reach about 30 people live on the phone. Of those 30 contacts, typically only 3 of them (one percent of the total 300) would qualify as a prospect interested in hearing about investment ideas from the firm down the road. This one percent success rate translates into a job where you spend a *lot* of time cold calling—something that I enjoyed less than a root canal with no anesthetic.

I completed the training program successfully and was now on my own. Having just spent the past six months telemarketing, I was desperate to find a better way to prospect for clients and rapidly build my business. Besides, I hated it when telemarketers disturbed me at home, so this was far from the fascinating aspect of Wall Street life that I'd envisioned at the start. Also, making a hundred phone calls to land one prospect seemed like an incredibly inefficient process.

If someone was interested in the stock market, I thought to myself, *couldn't there be a way to facilitate them finding me?*

While the Internet had been around since 1989, it wasn't until 1993, when the National Center for Supercomputing Applications (NCSA) at the University of Illinois Urbana-Champaign first introduced Mosaic, one of the first graphic user interfaces or web browsers, that it started to take off.[4] In 1993, there were approximately 2 million Internet-connected computers.[5] Nearly 25-years later, there are more than 3.5 billion Internet users that represent almost half of the world population.[6]

I had previously taught myself a variety of computer programming languages, such as C++, Pascal, and dBase, so I didn't give a second thought to learning HyperText Markup Language (HTML)—the programing language used for creating web pages and sites. Through trial and error, I created a functional website for Gruntal & Co. that provided visitors with basic information about the firm, market commentary, and an offer to receive a complimentary copy of the firm's investment ideas newsletter in exchange for the prospect providing necessary contact information and investment parameters.

At the time, none of the major full-service retail brokerage firms had launched their firm-wide sites on the Internet. The June 1995 issue of *Registered Representative*, a monthly magazine that was required reading for any stockbroker, was dedicated to The Information Highway, enticing readers with the caption "How to get on, stay on and find your way to 50 million prospects." Inside, I beamed with pride as I read that only "Two sites—one created by Michael D. Becker, a Gruntal broker out of Chicago, and the other, a site designed by Wertheim Schroder broker Thomas Gillespie in New York City—were blessed and endorsed by their firms."

The success of the website exceeded even my wildest expectations. People who asked for a free copy of Gruntal's investment newsletter were a stockbroker's dream—older, affluent individuals who bought stocks. Furthermore, every time a prospect completed the website form, I was immediately sent their profile information and alerted with an audible "You've Got Mail!" from my *America Online* dial-up account.

Thankfully, I never cold-called or telemarketed again. Now I could focus my attention on making clients money and building relationships.

———

On Friday, December 15th, 1995, I was at my desk reading the *Wall Street Journal* and having a coffee while the morning call broadcast from Gruntal's New York office over the loudspeakers. One of the firm's research analysts sounded more animated than usual, which caught my attention. He was talking about the dramatic reversal of fortune at struggling biotechnology company Centocor, Inc.—in particular, the company's positive clinical trial results that were announced after the market had closed the day prior.

In 1993, the FDA had declined to approve Malvern, Pennsylvania-based Centocor Inc.'s lead compound, Centoxin® (nebacumab), a monoclonal antibody for the treatment of sepsis, sending the company into a near-fatal financial tailspin and erasing an astronomical $1.4 billion from the company's market valuation. Adding to the company's woes, the slow ramp-up of Centocor's ReoPro® (abciximab) anti-platelet antibody to prevent blood clots from forming following FDA approval in December 1994 caught many on Wall Street by surprise. Some analysts had predicted first-year sales of the drug in the range of $70-$150 million. Instead, ReoPro sales for 1995 were less than $23 million.

Centocor's fortunes changed dramatically that day, however, and in retrospect, so did mine. The company halted a clinical trial of ReoPro after an interim analysis showed that it reduced death and heart attacks following balloon angioplasty procedures by 68 percent. The data were crucial for Centocor since it indicated the drug offered a strong benefit for the entire angioplasty market. Previously, the drug was only approved for the 10 to 30 percent of such patients considered at high risk of suffering a heart attack or other complications from the procedure.

Centocor's favorable trial results for ReoPro were a watershed event not only for the company but also for the entire biotechnology sector. The AMEX Biotech Index, which had been as high as 233 in November 1991, was at an all-time low of around 75 in March 1995. It would be the last time the index traded at such depressed levels.

Following approvals of Ortho Biotech's Orthoclone OKT3 in 1986 for transplant rejection, and Cytogen's OncoScint in 1993 for diagnostic imaging of colorectal and ovarian cancer, ReoPro was only the third monoclonal antibody-based product approved by the FDA. Its initial commercial failure had cast a long shadow on the field, but subsequent rise ushered a new era of important antibody product approvals. Today, monoclonal antibody therapeutics are one of the fastest growing, most successful, and lucrative segments within the biopharmaceutical sector.

Shares of Centocor's common stock rose $9 ¾, or nearly 70 percent, to close at $24 on the news that day. Regretfully, neither my clients nor I owned any shares of Centocor's stock at the time. Four years later, worldwide sales of ReoPro reached $447 million, and in mid-July of 1999, global pharmaceutical giant Johnson & Johnson announced that it would acquire Centocor for $4.9 billion, or $61.00 per share.

I was intrigued by a host of factors—the meteoric overnight rise in stock price, the market inefficiency, but most importantly, how to find the next Centocor. An investment opportunity that provided colossal upside *and* benefited human health? Undoubtedly there was no nobler financial pursuit. There was only one significant question left for me to answer: *What the heck is a biotechnology company?*

———

Super bull markets, those that span nearly a decade, have historically been once-in-a-lifetime anomalies, driven by extraordinary, life-changing technological transformations.[7] The 1920's super bull market, for example, fueled by the introduction of electricity into homes and factories, transformed lives and lasted nearly a decade before ending with the 1929 crash.

I've been fortunate to witness several super bull markets in my lifetime. The first was the 1990's super bull market that was fueled by the introduction of computers and automation. This bull market also gave rise to media-savvy "celebrity" analysts and strategists who had the power to move both markets and individual stocks through the views they expressed during television interviews on popular financial news networks.

I remember watching *Wall $treet Week with Louis Rukeyser*, a weekly television show that aired each Friday evening on public television in the United States from 1970 to 2002. The show attracted millions of viewers and has been credited with inventing the medium of investment broadcasting. Stocks mentioned by one of each week's special guest—mutual-fund portfolio manager, bank trust officer, economist—typically climbed the following Monday.

During the 1990's, Joseph Battipaglia served in many executive positions at Gruntal & Co. and frequently appeared on major media outlets in the national media, including CNBC, FOX News, and PBS' *Nightly Business Report*. Battipaglia's visibility was a great asset to new stockbrokers such as myself, as most investors recognized him and it added instant credibility when speaking to a prospective client on the phone. Sadly, he later died in 2011 at age 55 from a heart attack.

Each weekday during the noon hour, I watched CNBC as I ate lunch at my desk to hear the latest scoop from Dan Dorfman, a raspy-voiced Brooklyn native once dubbed the "nation's most prominent stock market tipster." Dorfman was hired by CNBC in 1990 after more than two decades of writing financial columns for the *Wall Street Journal*, *USA Today*, and other publications. As a business reporter, Dorfman appeared daily around noon on CNBC to offer his "pick of the day," a three-minute stock analysis that frequently included a buy or sell recommendation for a particular company.

As a stockbroker, you had to pay attention to Dorfman's daily picks. Invariably, clients would phone after the television segment aired to inquire whether or not they should act on his latest recommendation. Besides, there was a chance that some clients owned the stock being highlighted and it could be a natural pitch to take some short-term profits.

On November 3rd, 1995, however, I was focusing on a CNBC television interview with Liam Dalton, a portfolio manager at Axiom Capital Management in New York. He was bullish on Cytogen Corporation, saying the biotechnology developer had a "very good profile" and offered a "terrific risk/reward situation."

That day shares of Cytogen closed at $5 1/8, an impressive gain of more than 35 percent from the prior day's closing price. I didn't know its importance at the time, but that chance encounter with Cytogen would change my life forever.

I was deep into my research analysis of Cytogen by the time Centocor's favorable trial results were reported the following month. Immediately, I began noticing some of the similarities between the two biotechnology companies. Both were early pioneers in the monoclonal antibody space, both had marketed products that were underperforming Wall Street's expectations, and the stock prices of both companies were at the lower end of their historical trading range.

Having just witnessed the explosive upside of Centocor's stock, I began building a significant position in Cytogen for my clients. By early 1996, within just a few months, shares of Cytogen doubled, briefly touching $10—a multi-year high.

With the confidence of having started at Gruntal with zero clients and now having built a happy book of clients due to my website creation and Cytogen's strong performance, I decided the time was right to approach my father about returning to Wayne Hummer as a stockbroker. I reasoned that Wayne Hummer's Chicago heritage and conservative reputation would be a better long-term fit as my client base expanded. While the firm wouldn't have been a good match at the beginning of my career, the timing now seemed ideal.

Transferring firms can be a risky proposition. Stockbrokers at the old firm do their best to dissuade clients from moving their account to the new firm. It's akin to throwing chum in the ocean with sharks actively circling. Nonetheless, in the summer of 1996, I was welcomed "home" and rejoined Wayne Hummer as a broker. Fortunately, due to my close, personal relationships the vast majority of my clients loyally followed me.

The beautiful, windowed offices of Wayne Hummer were reserved for partners and large commission producers, so I was given a small cubicle and shared an administrative assistant with several others. As the chief financial officer for the firm, my father's office was on the floor below with rest of the operational staff.

Working at Wayne Hummer brought me closer with my father and his second wife, Linda. Being a partner and one of the firm's largest producers, Linda's client base was much larger than mine. She managed assets for high net-worth individuals, trust funds, and estates. Many of her customers had been with Wayne Hummer for years, and most of her new business came through referrals. As with my mother, Dad and Linda had met while working at Wayne Hummer, and they married in 1984. Linda's entire family was warm and welcoming to my sister and me from the first time we met. Linda's parents, Gloria and Casimir Kogut, were especially delightful.

With Linda's sister, Laura Kogut, and my uncle, Steve Becker, both partners at the firm, each day at Wayne Hummer was like a family gathering. By and large, business matters were kept separate from family issues and to the outside observer, you'd probably never know any of us were related.

I didn't have much interaction with Paul or Douglas upon my return, as they were still on the operations floor along with my father and Linda's sister, Laura. Now and then I'd see Douglas frantically running up the stairs and down the hall with "buy" or "sell" tickets for time-sensitive orders. At the time, brokers wrote their orders down on physical tickets and brought them to the order desk on the sales floor for execution.

———

In the summer of 1996, Lorie and I purchased a more substantial, three-bedroom, bi-level home in Skokie, Illinois. It was a short distance to the Old Orchard Shopping Mall, but more importantly, also near Jack's house. Lorie was very close with her family, especially her dad. When the weather was beautiful, particularly during summer evenings, the two of them would go for rides together in his Firebird convertible.

Due to hip and back problems, Jack enjoyed spending a fair amount of time laying horizontal on his oversized couch in the comfort of his own home. As there was little room for him to adequately sprawl in our house, we spent a lot of time there—especially after we had moved closer.

While I'm more into baseball, Jack was an avid basketball fan with Friday evenings reserved for gathering at his home to have dinner and watch the Chicago Bulls. After more than a year of "retirement" to try his hand at professional baseball, Michael Jordan had just returned to lead the Bulls back to another title in 1996. With an incredible supporting cast, including Scotty Pippen, the games were electric. I couldn't help becoming a fan. The Bulls not only took the NBA championship trophy that year but went on to win the next two, becoming just the third franchise in history to string together a trio of crowns.

Collectively watching the games throughout the seasons provided an opportunity to bond with Jack. Not only did we come to enjoy each other's company, but he also provided financial support to Lorie and I whenever needed. He was addicted to the stock market and opened a brokerage account with me at Wayne Hummer where he'd place more speculative bets, one of which included buying shares of Cytogen Corporation.

Unfortunately, the honeymoon with Cytogen was short-lived, as the stock soon declined from the double-digits and traded below the $5 level—where I had initially started buying.

I was surprised and disappointed by this downturn. It was also hurting my performance and reputation at Wayne Hummer. But it did provide great fodder for Jack, who enjoyed busting my chops every opportunity he got—and there were plenty.

"Where'd CYTO close today?" he'd ask with a sarcastic tone, already knowing the answer.

"Back where we bought it," I'd reply.

"Why didn't we sell it at ten?!" he'd shout jokingly.

"Sorry, my crystal ball has a hairline fracture."

I began to study Cytogen more carefully, conducting some in-depth research to find out why the company's stock was declining. On October 16th, 1996, I penned a terse letter to

Dr. Thomas McKearn, CEO of Cytogen at the time, expressing my disappointment with insider selling by one of the company's directors and the company's recent performance.

I wasn't the only one complaining about Cytogen's performance or lack of communication with its investors. Individuals flocked to the company's stock message boards on popular finance websites, such as Yahoo! Finance, to chastise management and complain about every downtick in the stock price. One particularly vocal nemesis went by the screen name "sick_of_this_stock" and took frequent jabs at management. Given my familiarity with Cytogen, several of these disgruntled investors initiated contact with me to discuss the company's prospects and ended up transferring their brokerage accounts to me. I informed them that while I was enamored with the company's technology and pipeline, Cytogen could do much more to increase its visibility.

One such investor was an eccentric dentist from New Jersey. Having made a fair amount of money with another biotechnology stock, he took passion and enthusiasm for Cytogen to new extremes. Convinced that it would be his next big winner and impressed by my knowledge of Cytogen and the general biotechnology sector, he transferred his sizable stock position in the company to Wayne Hummer. He encouraged nearly everyone else he knew to do the same. The dentist had a very kind heart and instructed all of his friends and family to invest in the company, hoping they would emulate his recent financial success.

As the size of my position in Cytogen increased, so did my interactions with the company.

———

In June 1997, Lorie's beloved pet bunny, P. J., died—about the same time Lorie found out that she was pregnant with our first child. We used the phrase "the rabbit died" to tell our parents and others that Lorie was pregnant, but few got the joke. The origins of the "rabbit test" go back to the discovery in the 1920's that a woman starts producing a hormone known as human chorionic gonadotropin (hCG) shortly after a fertilized egg implants itself in the uterine wall. Medical researchers found that not only is hCG present in the urine of pregnant women, but that female rabbits injected with urine containing hCG would, within a few days, display distinct ovarian changes.

Thus, the "rabbit test" was born, and with it the misconception that the rabbit's death was an indicator of a positive result. In those early days, the rabbit always died, because the animal had to be killed so its ovaries could be removed and examined. Fortunately, future refinements to the test enabled clinicians to inspect the ovaries without having to kill the rabbits first.

Up until the last trimester, Lorie's pregnancy was uneventful. I watched with amazement as her belly grew and my heart melted the first time I could feel our baby moving around inside. We took a local Lamaze class, which teaches parents healthy birth practices for safe childbirth and labor. Young, in love, and giddy with the expected arrival of our first child, we nearly got kicked out of class for laughing and disrupting the Lamaze group.

"I didn't know I was going into labor," the young mother in a training video the class was watching exclaimed. "I just thought that Philly cheesesteak sandwich didn't agree with me!"

Lorie and I made eye contact and immediately burst into hysterics. She got herself composed, but I loved to see her laugh and smile, so I started up again.

"Did that woman just say she mistook labor with indigestion?" I whispered in her ear. She started giggling again until the instructor "Shhh'd" us.

But towards the end of her pregnancy, Lorie developed high blood pressure and was restricted to bed rest. Eventually, even that wasn't good enough, leading to an artificial induction of the birth process through medical intervention. It was surreal *scheduling* your child's birth. I miss that I never got the frantic "Honey, I'm in labor!" phone call.

"I'm calling to arrange Lorie's induction," the scheduler at Evanston Hospital said to me on the phone. "The next opening would be Wednesday, February 4th, 1998 in the mid-afternoon."

"Okay, sure. That will be fine," I responded, sounding more like I was confirming a hair appointment or dentist visit instead of the birth of one's child.

After a casual lunch, we headed to the hospital that Wednesday for our childbirth appointment. After an overview of how the process would unfold, Lorie was connected to an IV and administered low doses of the hormone oxytocin to stimulate contractions and childbirth.

Lorie wasn't firmly committed one way or the other regarding the use of epidural anesthesia during childbirth, so we figured that it could be requested at any time during the process as appropriate. However, a few hours later, right about the time nurses changed shifts, Lorie was in a great deal of pain and requested an epidural. It took quite a while, but finally, she was comfortable as the anesthetic kicked in.

It seemed like an eternity of holding her hand and offering support throughout the hours of labor. Just before midnight, I watched as Lorie gave one last extraordinary push and our daughter entered the world crying and covered in goo.

"Would you like to cut the umbilical cord?" one of the nurses asked.

"Yes, please," I replied, nervously grasping the medical scissors from her hand and giving the last physical tie between Lorie and the baby a big snip.

The nurses whisked our baby to the pediatric scale tucked away in the corner of the delivery room. With only a knit cap on her head, she cried as the red LED numbers finally settled on six pounds, nine ounces. Considered full-term, but just on the edge—Lorie was induced early, and our baby appeared even smaller than I had envisioned. In contrast, I was the exact inverse of her weight at birth, topping in at nine pounds, six ounces. I was a big baby, as my mother always reminds me.

"So, Mom and Dad, what's her name?" the doctor asked us.

I knew Lorie wanted to name her after her mother, Rose. In Jewish tradition, there is a custom to name a child after someone, usually a family member, who has died. The usual explanation for this practice is that the parents hope that in receiving the name of an admired family member, the child will emulate in life the virtues of the deceased namesake.

It's also common for parents to alter or "modernize" the name of the deceased when given to the child. For example, only using the first letter of the relative's name. Another way to honor and commemorate through the name is to make a newborn child's middle name, as opposed to the first name, similar or identical to that of a special relative.

I wasn't overly keen on the name Rose, so we had compromised with the idea of using the first letter of her name. But after we'd been discussing various "R" names for a while, nothing had stood out. As I looked into Lorie's sparkling, but exhausted eyes, there was only one answer.

"Rose," I replied to the doctor, smiling at Lorie who nodded happily with my decision.

For her middle name, we chose Casandra, after Linda's dad Casimir, or Cas, who had passed away quite unexpectedly in March 1997 from a heart attack. We felt our newborn was getting doubly blessed being named after two such wonderful people.

A few days later, after visits from family and friends, Lorie and Rosie were released from the hospital. Lorie was in a wheelchair holding Rosie with a nurse while I went to retrieve our car. The baby's car seat was attached in the rear where I requested Lorie sit as well so she could monitor Rosie during the short trip home. As I walked away from them towards the parking lot, I began thinking. *How were we suddenly expected to be parents? Where was the instruction manual? What makes us qualified? Shouldn't we be required to pass some exam?*

During the ride home, I felt like everyone was aiming for our automobile, and more importantly, its precious new cargo. Driving well under the speed limit and encouraging frustrated motorists to pass, I carefully navigated the side streets of Evanston to our home in Skokie where we eventually arrived safe and sound.

Still feeling very unqualified for our newfound responsibility, especially when it came to taking Rosie out of the house, we nonetheless celebrated Lorie's Valentine's Day birthday the following weekend. We dined at a local restaurant with my father and Linda, with Rosie in her carrier and me nervous that a waiter would accidentally spill scalding hot soup on her—or something else terrible. I was an absolute nervous wreck.

But by the fall, I was feeling slightly more relaxed. We took a family trip with Dad and Linda to gorgeous Lake Louise, a hamlet in Banff National Park in the Canadian Rockies, known for its turquoise, glacier-fed lake ringed by high peaks and overlooked by a stately chateau. Using a baby backpack, Dad strapped Rosie on his back and proudly carried her as we walked the hiking trail up to the Lake Agnes Tea House for spectacular bird's-eye views of the area.

From day one, Dad and Linda were both proud grandparents, doting on Rosie and continually lavishing her with gifts. They enjoyed hiking and invited me to accompany them on the spectacular Iceline Trail located near Field, British Columbia in Yoho National Park. As a day hike, its steep ascent of about 1300 feet from the Takakkaw Falls parking lot to reach tree line—an eight-mile round trip—would be too much for Lorie and Rosie, so they stayed behind.

I wasn't in great physical shape and felt embarrassed that Dad and Linda were managing the hike much better than me. Climbing higher and higher, leaning more and more on my walking staff, I felt the burning in my legs. But the sublime views made up for any pain I felt.

I'd been afraid of heights since I was a kid, for reasons that are still not clear. Perhaps it was my first trip on Space Mountain at Walt Disney World as a child, which I vaguely recall other than it was terrifying. So, when we eventually came upon a tall pyramid of ground particles of rock, created ages ago by a glacier when the surrounding ice melted away, the walk to the top beckoned to me. I paused to study the width and height of the silt's edge, as I made up my mind to climb up the very narrow walkway leading to the peak.

"Are you sure you want to do this?" Dad asked me. He'd known about my fears when I'd refused to go on carnival rides and other high places in the past.

"Yes, I'm sure."

Seems like a good time to walk with purpose, I thought to myself.

Keeping my head down to watch where I was stepping, I slowly made my way across the ridge using my walking stick for balance when needed. Each time I put the stick down a miniature avalanche of rocks and pebbles slid endlessly down the large slope. Reaching the end, I looked down to behold the spectacular view from the top. Overlooking the gorge, I could see a melting glacier that fed a winding, turquoise river.

At that moment I felt empowered, albeit *terrified*, as there was scarcely more than one step in any direction before tumbling down the loosely piled rocks and pebbles that comprised the pyramid.

Unfortunately, I didn't conquer my fear of heights that day. However, I did learn something important about myself. Being able to walk that narrow path and reach the top was liberating. I rested for a moment at the peak to consider just how powerful one's mind can be. *If you want something bad enough, you can overcome nearly any obstacle.*

Being a fantastic photographer, Linda managed to capture a shot of me at the very moment I reached the peak. That image has come to represent my ability to walk with purpose and overcome obstacles. I glance at it often for inspiration. And while I'm still afraid of heights, I came away from the experience with a new love for hiking.

Chapter Four
Beck on Biotech

———

Due to the complex scientific and medical concepts, I found that I was spending significant time researching biotechnology companies and educating clients about the stocks that I was recommending for purchase. Explaining monoclonal antibodies, gene therapies, and signal transduction inhibitors to hundreds of retail investors was exhausting and time-consuming. I also wanted to leverage my rapidly expanding knowledge of the sector to attract prospective new clients that were interested in the field.

There must be a way to communicate biotechnology stock ideas more efficiently with my Wayne Hummer clients and prospects, I thought to myself.

Borrowing from Wayne Hummer's original concept of attracting customers by publishing its free market comment letters, I wrote up the inaugural issue of a monthly biotechnology-focused newsletter called *Beck on Biotech* in July 1998. Each month's edition provided an overview of a specific segment or aspect of the biotechnology industry along with a "company spotlight," a particular company that I was recommending to my clients. To track the performance of my spotlight picks, I also constructed a model portfolio.

Initially just one page (front and back), hard copies were printed and mailed to existing clients in advance of phoning them to discuss potential investment. This way, a client could review the company and its products in advance, so the phone conversation became much less time-consuming. Eventually, several clients would call me to place orders after receiving their issue in the mail. They also started sharing the newsletter with friends and family, which resulted in more new accounts and business.

Only after meeting with company's management or doing extensive due diligence would a stock make it into the coveted "company spotlight" section of *Beck on Biotech*. Companies could be removed from the model portfolio based on valuation concerns, clinical setbacks, or other potentially adverse developments. I also established a policy of only making additions or subtractions from the model portfolio with the publication of each month's issue.

Following years of lackluster performance, I found that many biotechnology industry executives were quite receptive to educating individuals such as myself about their company and products. Given the lack of quality analyst coverage and interested investors, my newsletter addressed an unmet need in the market by creating visibility for them. Accordingly, I had access to many senior executives in the sector that would not only take my calls but also fly to Chicago to visit with me face-to-face.

I couldn't take time to write each issue of *Beck on Biotech* during the weekdays since that's when I needed to focus on making sales. Instead, this labor of love would generally occupy the last weekend of each month.

"What are you going to write about in the first issue of the newsletter?" Lorie inquired over dinner one evening.

"The drug delivery segment of the biotechnology market—companies focusing on creating alternative delivery formats for drugs to address specific limitations in the market. For example, a company could convert a drug that had only been available as an injectable agent into a traditional oral tablet."

"And since many patients dislike needles, they'd take a pill with a sip of water if it were available."

"Exactly!"

"What company are you adding to the model portfolio for the first issue?"

"I found a company based in New Jersey named Enzon, Inc. Dr. Abe Abuchowski, a professor from Rutgers University, founded the company after discovering that coating a molecule with polyethylene glycol (PEG) could enhance its therapeutic properties by extending circulating blood life and lowering immunogenicity.

"And..."

"And using this new technology, they developed a new drug called Adagen® (pegademase bovine) for the rare genetic "Bubble Boy" disease. Adagen replaces an enzyme called adenosine deaminase that's absent from children who have the disease, so children suffering from the disorder can escape their sterile plastic environments and live relatively normal lives."

"Okay, that does sound pretty amazing."

Recognizing the need for a unified voice for the biotechnology companies of New Jersey, Dr. Abuchowski also established the Biotechnology Council of New Jersey (BCNJ), which was incorporated on January 26th, 1994. He was elected its first chairman and the organization started with 26 founding member companies, including Johnson & Johnson, Bristol-Myers Squibb, Enzon, Cytogen, and others.

Enzon became New Jersey's first biotech company to obtain FDA approval of a new product, but Dr. Abuchowski believed this technology could be used to improve the characteristics of many injectable and intravenous drugs.

Shareholders didn't have the same long-term vision or patience, however. So, in April 1994, Peter G. Tombros, a 25-year veteran with pharmaceutical giant Pfizer, was appointed the president and CEO of Enzon, while Dr. Abuchowski continued as chairman of the company.

Two years later, Dr. Abuchowski relinquished all of his responsibilities as an employee of Enzon and resigned from the board of directors. Its stock was trading just below $6 ½ despite the fact that Enzon was one of the few biotechs that had two drugs approved by the FDA and was generating revenue. I sensed the potential for a turnaround as Enzon transitioned from a company with significant losses to profitability. It earned Enzon the first company spotlight slot in *Beck on Biotech.*

Fortuitously, Enzon's stock turned out to be a fantastic start for my newsletter. The stock would ultimately be removed from the model portfolio in September 1999 at $33 ¾ per share, representing a gain of 424 percent in just over a year.

————

Meanwhile, things were not going well at all for Cytogen. By the summer of 1998, the company's stock price had declined below $1 and shareholders, like me, were quite upset. Sales of Quadramet® (samarium sm 153 lexidronam), the company's product to treat bone pain arising from cancer, were significantly below expectations, leading to a lawsuit and ultimate termination of a marketing agreement between Cytogen and DuPont Merck Pharmaceutical Company, the company's commercial partner at the time.

Reminiscent of the changes that had occurred at Enzon, Dr. McKearn relinquished his positions as chairman, president, and CEO of Cytogen and returned to a scientific role. He assumed responsibility as president of the company's Cellcor subsidiary, with the key assignment of seeking regulatory approval for Cellcor's Autologous Lymphocyte Therapy (ALT) that was being developed to treat kidney cancer. William C. Mills III, general partner of The Venture Capital Fund of New England and a member of the Cytogen's board of directors, assumed the role of chairman of the board. Another director, John E. Bagalay, Jr., was appointed interim CEO and an executive recruiter was hired to search for a permanent replacement.

With the company in such disarray, I made travel arrangements to meet with John Bagalay at the company's headquarters in Princeton, New Jersey on June 16th, 1998. It also provided me with an opportunity to attend Cytogen's annual meeting, which was taking place the following day. I was still fuming from my last visit, where I was informed upon arrival that Dr. McKearn was no longer CEO and that his interim replacement, John, wouldn't be able to meet with me due to prior engagements.

The next visit didn't go much better, as John was able to spend a short time meeting with me. After I quickly pointed out errors on the corporate slides he had prepared for our discussion, I was politely asked to "make some phone calls" in a vacant office while he conferred with other members of the management team. Nearly an hour passed when Jane Maida, the company's chief accounting officer and corporate controller, stopped in to see me.

"Any idea when John will be resuming our meeting?" I asked with extreme frustration.

"Unfortunately, John has a board meeting and won't be able to meet with you," she replied sheepishly.

My blood boiled but before I could even react, I was also informed that the names of people staying at the hotel, including myself and members of Cytogen's board of directors who had come from out of town, were posted on the company's stock message boards on the Internet and that the hotel received a bomb threat.

At this point, I had enough and made arrangements for a car service to return to the airport and head back home to Chicago. Upon my return, I penned another terse letter to Cytogen and awaited feedback on the outcome of the shareholder meeting.

Fortunately, Jennifer Fron Mauer, a reporter from *Dow Jones News*, covered the event and wrote a touching article about Bob Wegner, a 61-year-old man who spoke at Cytogen's annual meeting. Choking back tears, he talked about his wife, Mary Stamulakis-Wegner, whose breast cancer had spread to her bones, causing debilitating pain. Two weeks after her first dose of Quadramet, she was swimming and horseback riding again and "almost back to her normal self."

Wegner's story ended with a plea: "This product is great. Why don't more people know about it?"

The nearly 200 shareholders at the annual meeting burst into applause after Wegner's acute query. After reading the reporter's story, I felt reassured that I was correct about Quadramet's potential upside and awaited news on the company's promise to secure a new partner to market the drug and hire a replacement CEO.

On August 24th, 1998, Cytogen named Dr. H. Joseph Reiser president and CEO and as a member of the board of directors. Dr. Reiser's arrival at Cytogen coincided with a massive effort to turn around the company, which was running short on time and money. By the close of its quarter ending September 30th, 1998 Cytogen had only $3 million in cash left in the bank and was contending with the prospect of being delisted from the Nasdaq exchange due to its low stock price.

Joe moved quickly to rescue Cytogen, shutting down the cash-draining Cellcor subsidiary, eliminating one-third of the company's workforce, and curtailing research and development expenditures. He entered into a license agreement with Berlex Laboratories, Inc., a U.S. affiliate of Schering AG and his former employer, regarding the marketing of Quadramet, Cytogen's blockbuster-potential radiopharmaceutical product used to provide pain relief from cancer spreading to the bone. As consideration for the rights granted, Berlex agreed to pay Cytogen royalties based on net sales. Berlex also paid Cytogen $8 million in cash up front, of which half was used to secure a manufacturing agreement with DuPont Merck and to acquire from DuPont Merck rights to certain know-how and proprietary information related to the manufacturing process.

During the first year of launch, the company's previous marketing partner, DuPont Merck, had promoted Quadramet principally to nuclear medicine physicians. While those doctors typically administer radioactive treatments to patients, they are often first prescribed by care-giving physicians, including medical oncologists, radiation oncologists, and urologists. Not marketing the drug to the doctors who prescribe it meant that very few orders were placed. Cytogen believed that successful commercialization of Quadramet would depend upon selling to the essential referring physicians.

Confident that the outlook for Cytogen was improving, I knew it would take some time for Joe's turnaround efforts to bear fruit. Fortunately, my other biotech picks were performing well, which helped keep my retail client base happy.

———————

My career at Wayne Hummer was going well, although focusing on the risky biotechnology industry was a bit of a mismatch with the firm's conservative investment philosophy. Wayne Hummer also refused to encourage active trading in securities, but instead would foster a "buy and hold" investment strategy in the nation's strongest companies.

The client base that I had attracted were mainly speculators and traders looking to make quick profits. Despite my best efforts to diversify their portfolios by recommending blue-chip companies and mutual funds, this particular group of clients was drawn to the casino-like allure of Wall Street and couldn't be dissuaded otherwise.

Much to his chagrin, I became a frequent office guest of Elliott Silver, the firm's chief compliance officer. It was his job to ensure Wayne Hummer complied with all regulatory requirements, internal policies, and procedures. For example, soliciting the purchase of stock in companies not on the firm's approved list had to be approved by Elliott in advance. Also, each month's issue of *Beck on Biotech* had to be reviewed and approved by him before publication.

"Michael, I see you are adding Organogenesis, Inc. to your newsletter's model portfolio for an upcoming issue. Is the company making any money?"

"No, Elliot, they aren't profitable yet. But they do have a product on the market that is generating sales and the company should be profitable when they hit 100,000 units."

"How is their balance sheet? How long will their cash last them?"

"They have enough cash for about a year, but will need to raise more money."

"What does the company do exactly?"

"They're a biotechnology company making 'living' tissue-engineered products using cells isolated from neonatal foreskins. A recent issue of *Businessweek* named it one of the best products of the year."

"I'm sorry, did you just say *foreskins*?"

"Yeah. The product is constructed by culturing human foreskin from circumcised baby boys in a collagen matrix derived from cow fat. The foreskin is decontaminated with antibiotics, antifungals, and an ethyl alcohol rinse."

"Seriously?? And what do they use the product for?"

"The artificial tissue is used to promote the healing of chronic wounds, such as severe burns and diabetic foot ulcers. They have a large pharmaceutical partner marketing the product and it could be a multi-billion-dollar opportunity."

Elliott would continue asking questions until he was satisfied and even then, only begrudgingly sign-off on the issue.

"What do Ted and Linda think about all of this biotechnology stuff?" he asked.

"Well, they've never come out and said it, but I'm sure they would prefer that I spent less time researching biotech companies and more time following the firm's recommended list of conservative, blue-chip stocks," I replied.

Nevertheless, Elliott OK'd my continuing biotechnology pursuits. In fact, I think he was mildly intrigued and entertained by my analysis of the sector.

The timing for starting *Beck on Biotech* couldn't have been better. While most investors were focusing on Internet and related technology stocks, the established, bellwether biotech behemoths like Biogen, Inc., Immunex Corp., and Medimmune Inc. each ended 1998 with impressive triple-digit returns for the year. The first five companies added to my newsletter's model portfolio were also performing quite well. Enzon, which was the first company added in July 1998, had more than doubled by early 1999. Other additions, such as Chiron Corp., Affymetrix Inc., Alkermes Inc., and New Jersey-based Liposome Co., were also appreciating nicely.

But the newsletter wasn't just resulting in new brokerage clients and commissions; it also started attracting the interest of biotech industry executives seeking potential exposure for their companies. One such individual was Frank Baldino, Jr., who co-founded a biotech company called Cephalon in 1987 at the young age of 33.

I first met Frank at Wayne Hummer's office in Chicago, where he traveled from the company's headquarters in West Chester, Pennsylvania. Dark-haired and well-dressed, he exuded the warmth and outgoing nature of Italian culture that encourages the expression of emotions, which he often wore on his sleeves.

Frank invested significant time educating me about Cephalon, and to a lesser extent the broader biotech industry. The company was known at the time for its challenges in securing FDA approval for its lead product, myotrophin, which was being developed for the treatment of amyotrophic lateral sclerosis, or ALS, also known as Lou Gehrig's disease. Myotrophin showed efficacy in a U.S. clinical trial, but later showed no benefit in a European study. This uncertainty left the FDA in a quandary concerning approval, and the product's fate was still undecided at the time. Consequently, Cephalon's stock had declined significantly due to uncertainty over myotrophin.

Instead of belaboring the myotrophin outcome, however, Frank focused the majority of our discussion on Provigil® (modafinil), a pill that promotes wakefulness for the treatment of excessive daytime sleepiness associated with narcolepsy. Cephalon had acquired Provigil in February 1993 from Laboratoire L. Lafon, the French pharmaceutical company that first discovered modafinil.

The FDA had just approved Provigil in December 1998, and Frank walked me through the company's plans for commercialization and expected growth in advance of the product's launch in February 1999. He made convincing arguments for the wider use of Provigil beyond treating narcolepsy, including warding off fatigue in shift workers, multiple sclerosis patients, sleep apnea patients, and others.

Convinced of Provigil's upside, and equally impressed by Frank, Cephalon was the company spotlight for *Beck on Biotech's* first issue of 1999 when its stock was trading at $10 ½. Little did I know it would later become one of the best-performing stocks in my model portfolio.

Within a short period, *Beck on Biotech* amassed quite a following, with more than 1,000 individuals receiving a free copy of the monthly newsletter in the mail. With the February 1999 issue, the number of pages was increased from two to four, allowing more room to comment on the exciting biotechnology sector. Each new issue also included the following call-to-action:

"Beck on Biotech is a free newsletter which is provided as a result of the individuals who conduct their brokerage business with me.

If you find this information source valuable, it is my hope that you will place your trades with me in the future."

The newsletter also attracted members of the financial media looking for experts to interview as well as industry trade organizations looking for event speakers. Because of my coverage of several emerging New Jersey-based biotechs—Enzon, Liposome, and Cytogen—I was invited by Debbie Hart, president and CEO of BCNJ, to speak at their first networking event of 1999 at the Doral Forrestal Hotel (subsequently the Princeton Marriott) in New Jersey. Held on March 3rd, I viewed it as an excellent opportunity to network with industry executives and promote my newsletter outside of the Chicago market.

The hotel was located in the Princeton Forrestal Center, a 2,200-acre development project located a few miles north of Princeton University's main campus in Princeton, New Jersey. Beyond its six million square feet of campus-like office and research space, the Princeton Forrestal Center was home to other facilities and features, including hotels, conference centers, dining, and recreational trails and picnic areas. The John P. Moran Woods on the eastern portion of the project provided a network of scenic woodland trails covered with pine needles, walkways, picnic groves, and bicycle paths. The Delaware and Raritan Canal Park formed the western boundary.

Cytogen Corporation was among the project's 175 corporate tenants, which ranged from Fortune 500 companies to the smaller start-up firms. It provided an excuse to visit with Dr. Joseph Reiser and check on the company's turnaround progress following his arrival last summer. By this time, my Wayne Hummer clients represented an aggregate of approximately 500,000 shares of Cytogen, which started the year with its stock price hovering at $1. Joe had been very receptive to my calls and ideas since his arrival, and I thought it would be good to meet in person.

I had visited Tom McKearn, John Bagalay, and others at Cytogen's offices in the past, so I was quite familiar with the vast office complex. I was greeted in the lobby by Joan Greenjak, whom I knew from prior visits. She had been executive assistant to all of the company's CEOs over the years, going back to George W. Ebright, who was appointed Cytogen's president and chief executive in 1989.

"Hey you!" she said warmly followed by a hug.

"Great to see you," I replied. "So, how is the new boss treating you?"

"Very nicely, thank you. Let me take you back to his office. Can I get you anything—coffee?"

"No thanks."

Entering the corner office, I recognized Joe from his photos in various newspaper articles following his appointment as CEO. During our numerous phone conversations, I had noticed he was very guarded and concise with his words and sometimes could even come across as distant if you didn't know him better. He also had a slight German accent, since that was his native tongue.

"Dr. Reiser, it's a pleasure to meet you in person finally," I said, extending my hand to greet him as he rose from the chair behind the desk.

"Please, call me Joe. Won't you have a seat?" he replied, motioning to the small conference table in his office.

"You know, my wife and I spent quite a while in the Midwest when I was getting my degrees at Indiana University. It was quite nice there."

"Agreed, we like the Midwest a lot."

"Before we get started, I have meant to ask you. We're looking to fill a newly created position within the company for a vice president of investor relations and corporate communications. Have you come across anyone that you respect and think would be a good fit for Cytogen?"

"Yes," I said, pausing for a moment to run through the Rolodex in my head. "Right... I have come across quite a few in my travels, and there's one, in particular, that might be a good addition, Dr. Richard Krawiec. He headed investor relations and corporate communications at two companies I've covered in my biotech newsletter—La Jolla Pharmaceutical and Amylin Pharmaceuticals. I don't know him all that well, but he seems to know the science of biotech, having earned a Ph.D. in biological sciences. But he's based in California and might require a relocation package. I can reach out to him and see if he'd be interested since he seems to move around a bit."

"That would be great. Thanks for the suggestion. Would you like to go grab some lunch in the cafeteria and we can have a working lunch?"

"Sure, that'd be fine."

Over lunch, we discussed Cytogen's evolution into a sales-based organization, punctuated by his sale of the company's nearby manufacturing facility for $4 million and reduced expenditures in research and development. We also made pleasant small talk about stocks and other matters.

Shortly after our initial meeting, Cytogen and Progenics Pharmaceuticals, Inc. announced the formation of a 50/50 joint venture to develop vaccine and monoclonal antibody-based therapeutic products targeting prostate specific membrane antigen (PSMA). The protein is abundantly expressed on the surface of prostate cancer cells and is the molecular target for Cytogen's commercial product ProstaScint® (111In-capromab pendetide), a prostate cancer diagnostic imaging agent.

Earlier that year, Joe had promised to take significant action in advancing the company's PSMA target for therapeutic use. At the time, Progenics was a recognized leader in the area of cancer immunotherapy and could exploit PSMA on many fronts—including development of therapeutic antibodies and vaccines for the treatment of prostate and potentially other cancer types. Progenics already had two cancer vaccines in clinical trials: GMK to prevent relapse of malignant melanoma in pivotal Phase III trials; and, a second vaccine, MGV, under development for a variety of cancers, which was entering Phase II trials.

Convinced that the turnaround was well underway, I added Cytogen to the *Beck on Biotech* model portfolio with the August 1999 newsletter, with its stock price at $2. Although I had followed the company for quite some time, I was reticent to feature Cytogen in the newsletter until more evidence of the turnaround was in hand.

"With some major issues resolved, a more manageable rate of spending, and a dedicated management team," I wrote, "Cytogen is now better positioned to manage the marketing of existing products while looking for ways to enhance shareholder value."

Reporter Rob Garver with *Business News New Jersey* latched on to my bullish outlook for Cytogen, which was further bolstered by a fresh $5 million investment from the State of Wisconsin Investment Board, one of the world's largest pension funds and already a significant institutional holder of Cytogen's stock.

"While Becker's name isn't widely known, his spotlight portfolio has achieved impressive results since its inception in July 1998, achieving an internal return rate of 164 percent over the past 13 months," wrote Garver on August 9th, 1999. "Becker's track record with New Jersey stocks is even more impressive. He added Piscataway's Enzon to the portfolio on July 11 at $6.44 per share, and the company hit an all-time high of $27.00 last week. He added Plainsboro-based Liposome last November at $7.21. The company recently touched $28.50."

Little consolation for investors who'd purchased Cytogen's stock over the past few years, but with other picks like Enzon, Affymetrix, Liposome, and Cephalon up 296, 267, 283, and 83 percent, respectively, my brokerage clients remained quite happy.

———

As a result of the strong performance, I remained bullish on the sector's outlook and kept scouting for opportunities. I also continued advancing my career by becoming a Registered Investment Advisor after passing the Series 65 exam in January 1999.

During my interactions with Organogenesis, Inc., chief strategic officer Alan Tuck brought the biotechnology industry's overlooked roots in Illinois to my attention. When asked where biotechnology began, I naturally assumed that it had to be San Diego's "biotech bay" or somewhere in the "pharm country" of the East Coast. Much to my surprise, I discovered that the biotechnology industry could trace its success to my home state.

Former executives from three Illinois-based pharmaceutical giants—Abbott Laboratories, Baxter Healthcare, and Searle—helped create or lead more than a dozen elite biotechnology companies, including Amgen, Biogen, Genzyme, Gilead, Icos, Immunex, and Amylin Pharma. Collectively, these industry bellwethers accounted for more than 70 percent of the total Nasdaq Biotech Index market value and more than $5 billion in revenue at the time. With its rich history, I wondered why the state wasn't known as the biotech equivalent of Silicon Valley.

I quickly arrived at the conclusion that the industry languished in Illinois due to a lack of support from venture capitalists in the Midwest who were off doing Internet and dot-com-type funding that was viewed as less risky than their biotech counterparts. While the biotechnology sector started in earnest in the 1980's in areas like San Francisco and Boston, Illinois-based entrepreneurs complained in various local media outlets about their difficulty in raising capital to form new biotechnology companies in the conservative Midwest.

And then, there was the big fish that got away. Apparently in the early 1980's, chemist George Rathman and his California-based company, Applied Molecular Genetics Inc., wanted to build a major facility on Chicago's West Side to produce the next generation of genetically engineered pharmaceuticals. Although the $12-million project had substantial support from the administration of then-Mayor Jane Byrne and Governor James Thompson, a series of financing missteps slowed down and then scrapped the deal by 1985. Finally, after an unrelated change of direction in the company's production strategy, a 40,000-square-foot plant built for the company in the Chicago Technology Park went unoccupied.

While it was never the company's intention to locate its primary activities in Chicago, many employees at Applied Molecular Genetics (later named Amgen, Inc.) were Abbott alumni and would have liked to be located in the area. Instead, the company grew its business in California and became one of the leading biotech companies in the United States.

The presence of Amgen's manufacturing facility in Chicago could have dramatically altered the landscape and ignited a booming biotech industry in the region. Hoping to help reverse these trends, I became a founding member and director of the Chicago Biotech Network (CBN), a not-for-profit trade association in Illinois dedicated to assisting local biotechnology companies grow and promoting the industry in Chicago and the state. In 1999, I was invited to be the keynote speaker for the CBN's annual fall biotech investor conference, "Illinois BioMarketplace," which featured presentations by emerging Illinois biotech companies seeking corporate partners and investors.

To help create awareness for the Illinois BioMarketplace event, David Franckowiak, CBN's Treasurer, had convinced reporter Steve Ruxton at Chicago market television station WCIU to do a brief segment on the conference in advance. David's primary job was the CFO of Endorex Corporation, a local biotechnology company, and Steve had interviewed him previously about the company due to his role as business news anchor, editor, and reporter for WCIU. Steve hosted interview programs featuring guests in the areas of business, technology, politics and community affairs.

Marci Buettgen, CBN's president, had initially planned to join David for the television spot, but she ended up being under the weather that day. David asked me to stand in since I was the keynote speaker at the event.

It was my first time doing a live television interview, so I asked Lorie about it over dinner later that night.

"So, how'd I do on channel 26 today?" I asked her. "I was a bit nervous."

"It didn't show, and I was very proud of you. You made a lot of sense and didn't come across anxious at all."

"After a while, I felt like the reporter and I developed a good rapport."

"But I do think you need to grow your hair out a bit," she teased me lovingly. "It's too short and you know I like it longer."

My television debut proved quite valuable. I was soon invited as a regular guest and resident expert in the area of biotechnology. Coincidentally, another frequent guest on station WCIU was William "Bill" Hummer, one of Wayne Hummer's two sons who both followed their father in the banking and brokerage businesses. Bill's strong reputation as a financial advisor and chief economist at Wayne Hummer resulted in regular appearances in various local media outlets, including newspapers and two Chicago market television stations WCIU and WFBT.

––––––––––

Wall Street's attention had once again returned to the biotechnology sector in 2000, as evidenced by the surge in stock prices at the time. Investors were particularly enthusiastic about companies working to identify the greater than 100,000 genes that serve as the blueprint for all human life. Collectively, the genes are referred to as the "human genome," and the field of identifying each gene and its function is known as "genomics."

Although investor sentiment towards any company ending in "-omics" was analogous to the frenzy witnessed in the "dot-com" segment of the technology market, the enthusiasm appeared justified. Milestone events, such as the Human Genome Project sequencing chromosome 22 and Celera Genomics completing its human genome sequencing project later that summer, offered hope that they could revolutionize the way disease were diagnosed and treated.

On February 1st, 2000, enthusiasm for biotechnology stocks reached its zenith. The Nasdaq Biotech Index reached 1476, a level it would take more than a decade to recapture. With the sector in the spotlight, I knew that I couldn't afford to miss attending a large biotechnology conference that took place in New York City during the second week of February. However, I didn't relish the thought of being there in the winter like my prior trip for Kidder Peabody.

Unexpectedly, this visit to the East Coast proved far more beneficial. While preparing to leave my NYC hotel room and head over to the conference, my red Nokia 8210 mobile phone began to ring.

"Hello?" I answered, sounding confused. I wasn't expecting any calls.

"Is this Mr. Michael Becker, editor of the *Beck on Biotech* newsletter?" the woman on the line questioned. She sounded in a rush.

"Yes, umm, who is this?"

"I'm a producer with Bloomberg Television, and we'd like to do a live interview with you this morning regarding the biotechnology sector. Would you be interested and available?"

"Yes, that would be amazing!"

"Great, we're sending a car over to the conference hotel to pick you up now. Be downstairs in about 10-15 minutes. The car will have your name on it."

"Umm, okay," I responded as the line went dead.

To this day, I still don't know how Bloomberg got my cell phone number or knew I was in town for the event.

Waiting outside the hotel in the cold, I started to entertain the idea that the call was a hoax and that I was setup. Those thoughts evaporated quickly as the black town car pulled to the curb. In front of the driver's window was the name "Becker" written in black marker on a letter-sized piece of poster board.

After arriving at Bloomberg's studio, I was brought to a room to do hair and makeup. It was quite a different experience from my numerous appearances on the local Chicago cable television station. The makeup artist stuffed tissue paper between my neck and shirt collar as she applied powder to reduce shiny areas on my face and added a bit of color to my normally pale complexion.

Bloomberg television anchor Carol Massar met with me briefly to discuss the segment before we were escorted to the interview set. A microphone was attached to my lapel, and sound levels were checked. Then we went live.

"Joining me this morning is Michael Becker. He is the editor of *Beck on Biotech*. Good morning," the reporter started off the live interview.

"Great, thanks for having me."

"You write in your newsletter that we have all of the ingredients for a biotechnology revolution...how so?"

"Well, right now the industry statistics are all at record levels—you have a record number of products being approved by the FDA, a record number of products in the pipeline waiting for approval, you have more companies becoming profitable in the biotechnology industry than ever before, just about every industry metric is at a record level."

"Does this set it apart from the early 1990's when we saw a dramatic run-up in stock prices and subsequent fall back. Is it different this time?"

"I think it is. A lot of people thought back in the 1990's that it was going to be a quick process to get these products through FDA approval. People didn't realize that it takes $500 million and 15-years to get a product through the FDA approval process. Now it's 15-years later, and we have a flood of products in the later stages of development."

"Let's talk about a couple of the companies you like— Cytogen, La Jolla Pharmaceutical, Caliper, and Affymetrix. Right now, we're showing a graph of Cytogen, which had a dramatic run-up and most of them have a similar looking chart in the January-February time period. Tell us what's going on with Cytogen."

"Cytogen has recently come to the fore because they have a subsidiary focusing on an emerging aspect of the genomics industry called proteomics, or the study of proteins. That's really put the company into the limelight."

"And trading at $13—even though a stock like this is up 400 percent this year—you think there's still much more upside?"

"Actually, this was a company that traded at $30 in the early 1990's so you have to take a broader view of the biotechnology sector and remember what things were like then and how devastated the industry has been in recent years. And while the rebound has been dramatic, we're still not back at levels seen in the 1990's."

Following national television exposure, the little-known biotechnology stock called Cytogen became the fifth most-actively traded security in the markets on February 23rd, 2000 even as most investors scrambled to figure out its business.

———

The meteoric rise in the stock prices of many biotechnology companies resulted in a flurry of financing and banking activity. For an industry that raised only $5 billion in each year '96, '97, and '98, raising $12 billion in the first three months of 2000 was just astonishing. During the first quarter of 2000, the industry had its most significant private placement ever, plus its second largest follow-on. Nine biotech companies went public, collectively raising $1.1 billion—almost twice the amount raised by IPOs during the prior year.

Monoclonal antibody companies did exceptionally well at raising capital during this period. Abgenix raised approximately $454 million in a February 2000 follow-on financing. Medarex also tapped the public market, raising $359 million before the end of March in a stock offering managed by investment banks like Morgan Stanley Dean Witter, Chase H&Q, Dain Rauscher Wessels, and Warburg Dillon Read LLC.

Cytogen's stock continued to defy gravity, reaching nearly $22 per share in February 2000. Quite an improvement from trading below $1 just a short while ago!

At age 32, I owned nearly 24,000 shares of Cytogen for my brokerage account, which would be valued at more than $500,000 at its peak that month. Selling a portion of Cytogen's shares would have been the smart thing to do for both my clients and me. In such situations, however, greed tends to take control. I asked myself how much higher could it go? How much was all of the new genomic and proteomic data worth—especially if the key to solving major diseases was contained within?

Cytogen's market capitalization at the time was higher than $1.5 billion, but the value was being driven solely by the genomics bubble as opposed to improving fundamentals. In fact, sales of the company's commercial products were flat or declining, and cash levels were running dangerously low.

Nevertheless, the enthusiasm surrounding the Human Genome Project and Cytogen's plans to identify the first one million protein interactions made it difficult for me to step off the train. Through the company's AxCell Biosciences subsidiary, Cytogen expected to become the premier provider of proteomics data to the pharmaceutical and biotechnology market, with the launch of a database product by early 2001. Subscription revenue to the proteomics database was expected to establish AxCell as a profit center. Cytogen would also utilize the technology internally to discover and validate new drug targets.

However, the most significant challenge facing Cytogen wasn't being addressed: access to sufficient money to advance all of the company's ambitious programs forward to value inflection points. At the end of March 2000, Cytogen had approximately $12 million in cash and the company was still burning about $2 million per quarter. I urged management to follow in the footsteps of its monoclonal antibody industry peers and take advantage of the extraordinary funding window before it shut. With the company's value above $1 billion, raising $100-$200 million in return for selling 10-20 percent of the company's stock wasn't unrealistic.

But then on March 14th, 2000, U.S. President Bill Clinton and British Prime Minister Tony Blair released a much-publicized joint statement that was interpreted as preventing companies from filing patents on their raw genomic data, and the biotechnology stocks went into a tailspin, declining by 12.5 percent in one day. The overall Nasdaq index, which is heavily weighted with technology stocks, fell by 4 percent, its second greatest one-day fall ever at the time.

Here's what Clinton and Blair said: "To realize the full promise of this research, raw fundamental data on the human genome, including the human DNA sequence and its variations, should be made freely available to scientists everywhere…. Intellectual property protection for gene-based inventions will also play an important role in stimulating the development of important new health care projects."

It would be the last time Cytogen ever commanded a billion-dollar valuation.

———

Helping to distract me from the carnage in biotechnology stocks, in early 2000 Lorie was pregnant with our second child. By chance, it would be our first personal experience with biotechnology in action.

A routine triple screen maternal serum-screening test taken during pregnancy was found to be positive, indicating that our baby "could" have Down syndrome. We knew through conversations with Lorie's obstetrician and gynecologist, Dr. Susan Warner, in Evanston, Illinois, that this test offers the chance for a false positive.

To know for sure, we would need the standard method for detecting prenatal disorders (fetal karyotyping), which is a lengthy process that involves analyzing laboratory-cultured fetal cells (amniocytes) obtained from the mother's amniotic fluid through an amniocentesis. The whole process typically takes about seven to ten days to get results and, not being a very patient person, this seemed like an awfully extended period of anxious waiting.

Through my research of Illinois-based biotechnology companies, I had stumbled upon Downers Grove-based Vysis Inc., which developed, commercialized and marketed DNA-based clinical products providing information critical to the evaluation and management of cancer, prenatal disorders, and other genetic diseases. During 2000, the stock of Vysis closed as high as $19 ¼ and as low as $3 ½.

In late October 1997, the FDA had cleared for marketing the company's AneuVysion Assay, which was the first prenatal genetic test for Down syndrome and other chromosomal disorders associated with mental retardation and congenital disabilities. The test's 24-hour turnaround time seemed much more attractive than waiting 7-10 days with the older approach, so I told Dr. Warner about the newer test and she agreed to order it for us.

Fortunately, we received the results of the AneuVysion Assay within 24-hours as opposed to waiting more than a week, and they were negative for mental retardation and congenital disabilities. We were relieved.

Towards the end of the pregnancy, Lorie once again developed high blood pressure and induced labor was set for late in the afternoon on Wednesday, September 13th, 2000.

Lorie never struck me as a superstitious person, but she was quite upset with the prospect of giving birth on the 13th.

"It's not like it is Friday the 13th," I said, trying to lighten the mood.

"I don't care. I don't like the number 13 for a birthday. I prefer even numbers."

We arrived at Evanston Hospital and were escorted to our delivery room.

"I'd prefer to have my baby born on the 14th," Lorie pleaded with the nurse, "so anything you can do to slow down the process would be appreciated."

Like me, when she puts her mind to something, Lorie can accomplish just about anything. Sure enough, the nurse waited to break Lorie's water until midnight and a happy and healthy baby, Megan Elizabeth, was born hours later on September 14th.

Vysis was so enamored with our story that they later sent a team to our home to photograph our newborn along with Lorie and me, and our story was later featured in the company's annual report to stockholders.

"It was a huge relief when we received the results," Lorie was quoted saying in the company's annual report. "When the call came in on that Friday afternoon telling us everything was fine, I was so excited, I forgot to ask what sex the baby was...and had to call them back."

Vysis' diagnostic tests, which detect genetic changes in cells, gained a following among doctors, patients, and investors. One year later, the company was acquired by Abbott Laboratories for $355 million in cash or $30 ½ per share. Interestingly, while Vysis was mentioned as one of the few public biotechnology companies based in Illinois in the November 1999 issue of *Beck on Biotech*, the company never made it into the spotlight model portfolio. I didn't quite understand the value proposition of its products at that time. But now I sure did!

––––––––

In the May 2000 issue of *Beck on Biotech*, I suggested the spark that could reignite investor enthusiasm for biotech stocks was just around the corner. More than 20,000 participants would be gathering later that month in New Orleans, Louisiana for the year's largest cancer conference. Attendees of the American Society of Clinical Oncology, or ASCO, annual meeting exchange ideas and hear about the latest breakthroughs in cancer therapeutics and diagnostics from over 2,000 scientific abstract presentations during the four-day event.

It's no wonder that biotechnology industry observers closely watched ASCO. Entering the new century with 369 biotechnology products in human clinical trials—nearly half of them (175) for cancer—I reasoned that this year's ASCO meeting could be very rewarding to biotechnology investors.

The prior year, approximately 31 publicly traded biotechnology companies issued press releases regarding their presentation of new clinical data at ASCO. As a result, many of these companies witnessed dramatic appreciation in their stock price, which I dubbed the "ASCO-effect."

Doing my analysis for the newsletter, I studied the best-performing stocks from prior ASCO meetings held from 1996-1999 and noticed that many of the shares started to appreciate in *advance* of the meeting. I surmised this was due to the organization's policy of mailing abstract books to its many thousands of members about two weeks in advance of the start of its annual meeting, which is held every spring.

The books are chock-full of valuable research data from clinical trials scheduled for presentation at the meeting, and that is why many investors went to great lengths to obtain early access to them. It was clear to me and others that ASCO was facilitating the selective disclosure of potentially market-moving information to its members.

Due to a precipitous decline in the major biotechnology indices since mid-February's Clinton-Blair comment, I took the position in my newsletter that the "ASCO-effect" could be strong and swift in 2000. The newsletter highlighted some of the companies who could benefit the most from the upcoming ASCO meeting.

On May 19th, 2000, Carol Massar from Bloomberg TV did a segment regarding companies to watch at the upcoming ASCO meeting and quoted my newsletter and its "ASCO-effect" tagline.

It still bothered me that biotech stocks would rise or fall sharply as those investors "in the know" acted upon the data, while those not privy to the abstracts (like me) were left wondering why the stocks were moving. My ASCO-effect newsletter article caught the attention of Adam Feuerstein, a reporter with TheStreet.com at the time, who picked up the story and created additional pressure for ASCO to change how it disseminated abstracts for its annual meeting. In his article, Adam quoted one doctor who consulted for hedge funds as saying, "The first thing we did on April 10th was comb through the ASCO abstracts and start taking long and short positions. The information is a gold mine...especially for those that are medically sophisticated."

Amazingly, a new abstract distribution policy wouldn't be put into place until the 2008 ASCO annual meeting. Under the new system, about two weeks before the start of the meeting, ASCO mailed research abstract books to its members, as it had always done. But at the same time, the research abstracts were posted on the ASCO website, fully accessible and searchable by anyone. Investors no longer had to worry that people were trading on information that wasn't publicly available.

"Making the abstracts available to the general public two weeks prior to the meeting, as opposed to selectively disclosing them only to ASCO members, would level the playing field and be consistent with the spirit of Regulation FD. Such a relaxation of embargo policy is long overdue and a welcome change," I said during one media interview.

Indeed, leveling the playing field was a significant milestone in helping add transparency and simultaneous disclosure of information to all investors.

———

By the summer of 2000, Cytogen's cash had further declined to just over $10 million, while product sales remained below Wall Street's expectations. Much to my chagrin, the company didn't raise any significant capital during one of the largest biotechnology funding windows in recent memory. Instead, on July 10th, 2000, I received a copy of a joint press release from Cytogen and Advanced Magnetics, Inc., announcing that they had entered into a merger agreement under which Cytogen would acquire Advanced Magnetics, a developer of novel contrast imaging agents used with MRI to aid in the diagnosis of cardiovascular disease and cancer. Under the terms of the acquisition, Advanced Magnetics' shareholders would receive $60 million in shares of Cytogen common stock.

As I finished reading the lengthy press release, my office phone rang.

"It's Dr. Reiser from Cytogen," my assistant, Tracy, said. "Shall I put him through?"

"Yes, please."

"Good morning, Michael. I assume you saw our press release issued just now?" Joe said upbeat and confidently.

"Yeah, I saw it."

"You don't sound very enthusiastic?"

"I'm not, as I would have preferred to read that Cytogen raised much-needed capital. Acquiring Advanced Magnetics sends investors a lot of mixed messages."

"How so?"

"Well, Cytogen was supposed to be transitioning away from diagnostic and imaging agents to focus more on lucrative therapeutic products. But now you've bought a company that expands your diagnostic and imaging franchise. Also, one of your early actions was to sell Cytogen's manufacturing facility to get out of that side of the business, but now you're buying a company with a manufacturing facility. And although you're getting close to $20 million in cash and marketable securities through Advanced Magnetics, the combined company will still be undercapitalized and need to raise more money. I'm not sure investors will react favorably to the news."

It was the first time that I disagreed outright with one of Joe's decisions, but he listened carefully to my points and concerns. Nonetheless, he was quite optimistic about the prospects for Advanced Magnetics' near-term product opportunity, Combidex® (ferumoxtran-10), an MRI contrast agent designed to aid in the detection of lymph node metastases. The product candidate had produced promising clinical results, and the FDA had recently issued an "approvable" letter for Combidex following a priority review. Advanced Magnetics was developing another product, ferumoxytol (Code 7228), for use in oncology applications as well as MR angiography.

Sure enough, the day that the merger was announced, shares of Advanced Magnetics, based in Cambridge,

Massachusetts, rose $1.81, or almost 30 percent, to close at $7.88, while shares of Cytogen fell $1 ¾, or 15 percent, to close at $9.56.

Joe and I continued a spirited debate about the pros and cons of merging the two companies following the announcement. However, what I didn't appreciate at the time was that Cytogen's introduction to Advanced Magnetics came via one of its board members, S. Leslie Misrock, a New York lawyer who was an authority on biotechnology patent law. He was a senior partner in the Manhattan-based law firm of Pennie & Edmonds and represented many biotechnology companies. He was also a prostate cancer survivor.

Leslie knew Jerry Goldstein, CEO of Advanced Magnetics, who founded the company in November 1981 and completed its initial public offering in June 1986. Leslie and Jerry were much more sanguine about ferumoxytol as a blockbuster *therapeutic* product for iron-replacement treatment in people with kidney disease. Unfortunately, this key message wasn't communicated at all as part of the merger announcement.

Advanced Magnetics' product portfolio consisted of iron-based products that affect the MRI signal properties of surrounding tissue. These contrast agents are used primarily to increase the sensitivity of MRI. However, the human body also needs iron to produce healthy red blood cells or hemoglobin, which carries oxygen through the bloodstream. If your body doesn't have enough iron, such a deficiency can cause anemia, which means that you have too little hemoglobin.

A key feature of Advanced Magnetics' ferumoxytol was its ability to be administered in larger doses than existing iron replacement therapies. Ferumoxytol was also supposed to be more convenient for patients because it could be administered at their doctor's office rather than an infusion clinic.

Succumbing to stockholder pressure, Cytogen announced via a press release on August 28th that it had canceled plans to acquire Advanced Magnetics but had instead entered into licensing, marketing, and supply agreements for the rights to two Advanced Magnetics products in exchange for two million shares of Cytogen common stock and royalties based upon future product sales. Cytogen received exclusive U.S. rights to Combidex—the product that Joe was excited about, and also the imaging agent ferumoxytol for oncology applications, plus the right of first negotiation for applications outside of oncology, such as its blockbuster potential as an iron-replacement therapy. Advanced Magnetics retained responsibility for all costs associated with clinical development, supply, and manufacture of the products.

Under the terms of the "new" agreement with Advanced Magnetics, the two million shares of Cytogen stock they received were valued around $16 million if sold at the prevailing market price around $8 per share at the time.

Under the terms of the agreement, 500,000 shares were held in escrow pending the achievement of certain milestones relating to Combidex and ferumoxytol. The remaining 1.5 million shares were transferred to Advanced Magnetics and could only be sold into the market at a rate of 300,000 shares per month. While this avoided the immediate potential of having 1.5 million shares being sold by Advanced Magnetics, I feared it could still create steady, downward pressure on Cytogen's stock over a five-month period.

The deal was a lot smaller than the planned acquisition that had been scrapped, and Advanced Magnetics' holders were not happy. Cytogen shares declined modestly the day after the new deal was announced, falling 1 percent to close at $8.94. But Advanced Magnetics' stock lost nearly one-third of its value, dropping $2.44 to close at $5.13.

Cytogen's rights to ferumoxytol for other indications, such as iron replacement therapy, were predicated on Advanced Magnetics first requesting a proposal from Cytogen and then Cytogen notifying Advanced Magnetics in writing within five business days after receipt of such notice of its interest in obtaining such rights. Apparently, such a proposal was made, but Cytogen didn't respond within the allotted 5-day time period, thus forgoing rights to the lucrative iron replacement market.

By December 2000, uncertainty over the Presidential election, rising oil prices, disappointing corporate earnings, continuing conflict in the Middle East, a weakening European currency, and end-of-the-year tax-loss selling had contributed to further declines in stock prices. Shares of Cytogen's stock, which had never recovered from the botched merger with Advanced Magnetics, continued to drop even as the company announced a new marketing agreement with Canadian pharmaceutical company Draxis Health, Inc. to market the company's advanced iodine-125 and palladium-103 "BrachySeed" radioactive seed implants, or brachytherapy products.

At the time, brachytherapy was a fast-growing therapy for early-stage prostate cancer and offered some potential benefits compared to alternative treatments such as radical prostatectomy, including rapid patient recovery, lower costs, and reduced incidence of complications such as impotence and incontinence. Independent estimates at the time placed the U.S. brachytherapy market at more than $200 million.

In contrast to the Advanced Magnetics' deal, entering the brachytherapy market made a lot more sense to me. First, it was an established *therapeutic* market and Cytogen appeared to have a differentiated product to offer. Second, radiation-based products were within Cytogen's core competency. Lastly, there was also an opportunity for cross-selling with its approved prostate cancer imaging agent, ProstaScint.

Nonetheless, after trading as high as $21.81 at the start of 2000, Cytogen's stock ended the year at $2.00 per share. I was interested to see that the bulk of the decline occurred in the same period when the 1.5 million shares were transferred to Advanced Magnetics and dismayed that my reservation about Cytogen's stock coming under selling pressure was validated.

Chapter Five
Leaving Wall Street

The year 2001 started off with a bang in the one-story building near a cornfield in eastern Bucks County, Pennsylvania, headquarters for Cytogen's AxCell Biosciences subsidiary. AxCell announced the completion of the first-ever map of a human protein family, representing a significant milestone in its efforts to chart all protein interactions. When completed, a map of protein interactions could play a role in pharmaceutical developments by helping identify drug therapies that target disease more effectively and with fewer side effects.

Using advanced robotic screening techniques and data made available through the Human Genome Project, AxCell scientists successfully identified more than 69,000 different protein interactions of the "WW domain," the name for one of the human body's 60-80 specific domain families. A domain is a structural site on a protein where interaction occurs with another protein.

Because protein signaling pathways play a role in many diseases, scientists are working to develop drugs that specifically target these pathways. While some interactions are likely to have positive clinical results, others can lead to unwanted drug side effects and toxicity. By referring to a chart of the body's protein interactions, researchers may be better able to identify drugs that target pathways related to a specific disease while avoiding those pathways associated with unwanted side effects.

Commenting on the achievement was Leroy Hood, M.D., Ph.D., an American biologist and president, co-founder of the Institute for Systems Biology, and one of the earliest advocates of the Human Genome Project. The inventions developed under his leadership include the automated DNA sequencer and an automated tool for synthesizing DNA.

"AxCell has provided an interesting dataset for understanding protein signaling pathways," Dr. Hood was quoted in the company's press release. "This achievement, a systems analysis of the WW domain family, provides important new information on protein signaling pathways which could have implications for their role in a broad range of diseases."

In advance of the news release, Linda A. Johnson, a reporter for The Associated Press who was doing a story on AxCell's accomplishment, contacted me on the phone. I was quoted in her article:

"I think the mapping of the protein domains is of equal or greater importance to the drug development industry than sequencing the human genome."

Driven by this achievement, Cytogen's stock was once again catapulted into the limelight and its stock price more than doubled, rising from $2.66 to close at $5 3/4 on Friday the week AxCell's news came out.

During a congratulatory phone call, Joe again asked if I knew any good investor relations professionals to recommend.

"Richard barely lasted one year before leaving to join Progenics," he said.

"Yeah, I do feel bad about that. But given my familiarity with the company, perhaps I should just come onboard and do the job myself," I replied.

I was half-joking, but the words left hanging for a moment, giving us both pause.

"Well, you do owe me one after that last recommendation."

"Indeed. OK, I'll ask around and let you know if you I find anyone."

After we hung up the phone, I started to seriously think about the prospects of joining Cytogen and leaving Wayne

Hummer behind. I was already nervous about the overall stock market and the impact a prolonged bear market would have on my commission-based business.

Earlier that week, Linda had shared a market newsletter making the case that after outsized returns during the latter part of the 1990's, investors should have realized that returns and valuations were unsustainable. Essentially, the above average returns during the 1980's and 1990's could be viewed as having been "borrowed" from the decade starting in 2000. In the 1980s and 1990s, for example, large company stocks averaged annualized returns of 17.6 percent and 18.2 percent, respectively, well above historical averages of approximately 10 percent. By some estimates, it could take a decade of subpar stock market returns to restore balance.

When I initially left Wayne Hummer to join Kidder, Peabody & Co., I was single and had arrived at a decision entirely on my own. This time, there was far more at stake, including a wife and two young daughters. I decided later that evening, after the kids were asleep, that it was time for another "talk."

"I read an interesting article today at work," I started off gingerly.

"About what?" Lorie responded.

"Basically, saying that the stock market could underperform until 2010."

"Oy! What would that mean for you as a stockbroker?"

"Well, they say there's money to be made in both bull and bear markets, but I'm worried that clients are getting too greedy. I've been getting a lot of pushback when I try to recommend diversifying into more defensive sectors, such as gold."

"So, what are you thinking of doing?"

"I spoke with Joe, the CEO at Cytogen, and he was asking for another referral to head up their investor relations department. It got me thinking—I mean, clearly, I know the company and its technology quite well. And having a financial background along with the scientific knowledge I've gained over the years writing my biotech newsletter could be a real asset. Besides, I seem to get along pretty well with Joe."

"Wow." She digested the news. "You've hinted at the idea in the past, but I still didn't expect it. You definitely know the company quite well. Would we have to move to New Jersey?"

"I haven't approached Joe about the idea formally, so there are a lot of details to be worked out—if he's even interested. But the company did pay to relocate the last hire, so I'm sure that would be a consideration."

"But everyone we know is here in Illinois," she said despondently.

I knew the idea of moving across the country would be the hardest for Lorie, especially leaving her dad. All of our friends and family were local as well, including Lorie's support network, who were so important when Lorie was confined to bed rest during both pregnancies. Who would be there for her when I'm at work and she didn't know anyone for nearly 800 miles? And what about how Lorie's dad was getting older—what if he got sick and needed her help? Nevertheless, I wanted to keep the idea alive and at least see if we could make it work.

"I think this could be a positive for our family," I said. "If nothing else, we can consider it an adventure and try it out for a few years. If we don't like it, we can always come back to Chicago. Who knows, maybe by then the biotechnology sector will finally be booming in Illinois."

"You know how commissions and the uncertainty of every month's paycheck stresses me out," Lorie said. "Having a regular paycheck again would be nice. If you think it's the right thing for our family, you know that I'll support you."

"To be fair, I have developed a pretty good track record. Leaving computer programing to become a stockbroker worked out pretty well. And leaving Gruntal to join Wayne Hummer also went smoothly."

I was in my early thirties, had a mortgage, two young daughters, and a rising Wall Street-focused career. I was the third-generation member of my family to work at Wayne Hummer where I'd established myself as a successful portfolio manager and securities analyst. I knew staying at Wayne Hummer would be a right long-term decision, especially given my family's history there. But I believed in Cytogen and its cancer product portfolio enough to warrant taking a risk.

I spoke with Joe several times over the phone as we ironed out the details of my employment offer. It was a generous package that offered more income than I would reasonably expect to earn in the brokerage industry during the coming years—especially during a bear market. Most of the relocation expenses were covered, and there was also a bonus and stock incentive plan. I would receive an auto allowance, an office, and a dedicated assistant.

I decided to take the plunge.

————

Arriving at Wayne Hummer the next morning, I asked to meet with Dad and Linda. My father offered to meet us in her office, as Linda and I were both on the sales floor. Once he arrived, I began to tell them the big news.

"I know this is going to come as quite a shock, but Cytogen offered me a position with the company. I've given it a great deal of thought and know that in the long-run there might be more upside by following in the family's footsteps and possibly becoming a partner at Wayne Hummer. However, with the negative market outlook and now having two extra mouths to feed, I've decided to take the job and move to the East Coast."

Not surprisingly, they were both wholly stunned, and it took a moment for them to process the news and its vast implications.

"Michael, first of all, congratulations," Linda was the first to speak. "We know that you will succeed at anything you put your mind towards."

She was always supportive of me and the first to offer positive reinforcement.

"What is your position with the company?" my father asked.

"Vice president of investor relations."

"Please don't take this the wrong way, but just how financially sound is Cytogen?" Linda astutely asked.

"They have enough cash to last maybe a year, so they will need to access more capital. That's one of the areas where I think that I'll be able to add some real value."

"How soon will you be moving?" my father asked.

"They are quite flexible, so I can commute for a few months from Chicago while we look at homes and decide where we want to move."

It was a lot for them to absorb, so the initial conversation was brief. Later on, I discussed my desire to transfer all of my clients to Linda instead of distributing them among various newer brokers, and she agreed.

"I'll create a letter to send out to all my clients letting them know about my move and that you'll be handling their accounts going forward," I told her. "For the larger accounts, we might want to have a brief teleconference to address any questions and ensure a smooth transition."

"Okay, but you're going to need to help me with all those biotechnology stocks," she replied. "I might be calling you frequently with questions about them."

"Of course, I'm happy to help."

With the benefit of hindsight, after the technology bubble burst in 2000, from December 2000 to December 2010 the S&P 500 index delivered an annualized return of just 1.2 percent, underperforming both T-bills and treasury bonds. It would have been a challenging period for a relatively new broker such as myself.

Among the many difficult outcomes of leaving the financial services industry was closing my *Beck on Biotech* newsletter. I enjoyed researching and writing about the sector, but March 2001 represented the final newsletter issue. The model portfolio's internal rate of return from July 31st, 1998 through February 28th, 2001 was 397.40 percent compared with a 329.08 percent return for the AMEX Biotech Index during the same period. Cephalon was one of the biggest winners, up 448 percent to $57 ½ as of the last issue. Other strong performers at the time included Alkermes, up 326 percent to $31, and Chiron, up 178 percent to $47.19.

———

A few days after accepting the employment offer for Cytogen and resigning from Wayne Hummer, a package arrived in the mail at home. It was from Cytogen, and the contents were various new employee forms for me to complete and return to the company's human resource department.

As I went through them—health insurance forms, tax withholding, 401(k) plan—I came across one that was potentially problematic: college transcript request form. On my resume, I had listed "completed coursework" at DePaul University from 1991-1995. I just assumed that everyone knew "completed coursework" was code for "no formal degree obtained."

"I'm seriously uncomfortable with this," said Lorie after I briefed her on the situation to get her perspective.

"Me too, especially in an industry where education is so highly valued. Could it be that Joe assumed I had a college degree? Or maybe he didn't look closely at my resume?"

"Could he rescind the job offer after learning that you don't? Or what if it doesn't come up for weeks or months down the road—or after we've already moved?" Lorie asked concerned.

"Maybe he knows that I don't have a degree and he believes that my career speaks for itself. Let's face it, with all of the financial exams I've passed and after reading my biotech newsletter; he knows by now that I'm not some idiot."

"You simply have to call him," Lorie stated bluntly. And, of course, I knew she was right.

Lorie sat at the long end of the sectional sofa in our family room as I nervously paced the beige carpet listening to the phone ring. She stared sympathetically at me the entire time, knowing how challenging it was to make the call. I had already begun to leave Wayne Hummer, so a vital career opportunity hung in the balance. Finally, Joe picked up.

"Good evening, Joe, I hope I'm not disturbing you, is this a good time to talk?" I said with my voice already cracking from nerves.

"Sure, no problem. What's on your mind?"

"I just got the employment paperwork from human resources, and there is one issue that I want to clarify with you."

"What's that?"

"There's a college transcript form included in the packet. On my resume, I listed 'completed coursework' at DePaul University from 1991-1995, which of course is true. However, I never got a formal degree and didn't want to get off on the wrong foot by having any misunderstanding."

It was clear from the long pause that followed that Joe wasn't aware that I didn't graduate from college. Lorie could sense my apprehension and she looked panicked. Not by what the outcome meant to us as a family, but because she knew what it meant to me personally and how it was eating me up inside.

"Thank you for the clarity. In fact, I wasn't aware," Joe paused again. "However, this won't affect our plans and I appreciate your transparency on the topic."

"OK, Joe...Thanks," I said, with a great sigh of relief. "I'll fill all the paperwork out and send it back to HR. Looking forward to getting started."

I am eternally grateful to Joe for the trust he placed in me at that moment. As I gave Lorie a big hug in relief, I started thinking about one of my biggest regrets in life—not attending college right after high school—and how it could have just derailed a promising career opportunity. But, between managing work and raising a family, it was becoming more and more challenging to find time to take classes and continue pursuing a degree in the evenings.

One thing was sure: I would strongly encourage my daughters to obtain a college when the time came.

———————

The press release announcing my new role at Cytogen crossed the newswires on Monday, April 9th, 2001. One of the first people to phone me was Frank Baldino, Jr. from Cephalon.

"I had no idea you would entertain the idea of joining a biotech company and relocating," he said on the phone. "You must come work at Cephalon instead. What did they offer you? We'll beat it."

"I'm flattered Frank, and the concept only surfaced recently. It didn't even occur to me that you might be looking to fill an investor relations position. Unfortunately, I made a commitment to Cytogen and the press release is already out. So..."

"Nonsense, this is business and things like this happen all the time," he cut me off. "Let's have lunch and by the time we're done, I'll have you convinced. Are you in town this week?"

"Yes, I am."

Frank took me by surprise and I knew it would be difficult, if not impossible, to go work for him—especially given Joe's trust in me and already joining Cytogen. But I confess to having been flattered and somewhat curious, so I went along.

"Great, I'll have my assistant make a reservation at the Peacock Inn near you in Princeton, New Jersey."

Arriving at the restaurant a few days later, it was clear that Frank frequented the establishment. He conversed with the host, and we were shown to his favorite table.

Through our many meetings and conversations over the years, I had come to appreciate that Frank did not like failure. He always liked to win—even cheating at golf.

"Thanks for agreeing to meet on such short notice," he started. "Look, we need someone like you in the investor relations position at Cephalon. You have a very different background, understanding both the science and financial aspects of our business."

"Frank, you know that I have the utmost respect for you and everything that Cephalon has accomplished. Adding your company to my newsletter's model portfolio around $10 per share made it one of the best performers among my picks. And..."

"And we have much farther to go," he interjected. "I want you to give serious thought to joining the company. Why don't you come by our corporate headquarters and at least meet some of the team?"

"Sure, I'd like that," I replied, hoping that gesture would be enough to satisfy Frank's desire to win.

"Let's change subjects. Have you started looking for a home? Where are you thinking of relocating?"

"We've been researching the Bucks County, Pennsylvania area..."

"You know there are some great places near West Chester," he interjected, making a subtle plug for joining Cephalon.

"How do your parents feel about you moving?" Suddenly his tone shifted from hard sell to genuine concern and interest.

"They're supportive, but not seeing their two granddaughters as often will be the hardest part for them. My dad and step-mother both work at Wayne Hummer, and we'd all go out for dinner at least once a week."

"Step-mother?"

"Yes, my parents are divorced."

"How old were you when they got divorced? Did your mother also remarry?"

"I was 12-years old when they divorced. My dad remarried a few years later. My mother remarried in 1997."

"You know I just got remarried. It's been tough for our three kids from my first marriage. How were you impacted by the divorce?"

I remember thinking at the time that the conversation was taking an odd turn. But Frank seemed to be seeking reassurance that, with the passage of time, life with his children could return to normal.

"The divorce was tough, but I never resented either of my parents. It took some time to adjust, and I'm sure your kids will too."

After the lunch, I scheduled a subsequent visit to Cephalon's offices in West Chester, Pennsylvania as Frank suggested. Later that evening, Lorie and I debated the opportunity, but we agreed that entertaining a job offer from Cephalon wasn't appropriate at the time. I felt that it was prudent to maintain the relationship—especially if things didn't work out well for Cytogen down the road. As a result, I planned on moving forward with the scheduled meeting. Besides, Frank wasn't going to let go easily.

It was about an hour drive between Cytogen and Cephalon. I decided to visit the next time I flew to Philadelphia International Airport and drove directly from there since it was closer.

Cephalon's offices were quite impressive, reflecting the fact that the company was generating nearly $50 million in quarterly sales and had approximately $100 million of cash in the bank. The company employed more than 1,100 individuals, with about half located in the United States and half in Europe.

Frank had arranged a tour of the 160,000-square foot office and research facilities. He also scheduled interview rounds with key staff, including Kevin Buchi, CFO, Carl Savini, senior vice president of human resources, Sheryl Williams, senior director of product communications, and others. One thing became clear from each of the meetings: Cephalon's strong stock appreciation had cultivated many wealthy and loyal employees.

Undeniably, Cytogen and Cephalon were very different companies at very different points in their life cycles. I couldn't help wonder if Cephalon, having already become a success, perhaps lacked the same upside potential as Cytogen. Then again, Cephalon was much more financially stable than Cytogen. It was an interesting crossroad.

In the end, my integrity and commitment to Joe prevented me from abandoning Cytogen, despite the generous offer Frank had extended to me. A decision that Lorie fully supported.

———

One of my first tasks as an official employee at Cytogen was among the more memorable. To help the company's AxCell Biosciences subsidiary, board member S. Leslie Misrock, Esq. had once again made a valuable introduction to a potential business partner, Cadus Pharmaceutical Corporation.

Cadus, formerly a biotech company engaged in research and development until it sold all research assets to OSI Pharmaceuticals in July 1999, was noteworthy less for its science and more for one of its significant stockholders, billionaire Carl C. Icahn, an American investor and business magnate who developed a reputation as an activist investor and corporate raider. Icahn initially invested in Cadus in a private financing in 1993.

Following the introduction from Leslie, Cytogen had been working with Russell Glass, who served as the president and CEO of Cadus, to explore potential synergies between Cadus and AxCell Biosciences. In addition to his role at Cadus, Russell was president and chief investment officer of Icahn Associates Corp., a diversified investment firm, which meant Icahn was ostensibly his boss at the time.

Cadus had developed proprietary yeast-based drug discovery technologies that were potentially complementary to AxCell's proteomics platform. I worked on preparing documents and slides to help demonstrate the synergies between the two companies in advance of Russell presenting a proposal at an upcoming Cadus board meeting.

In preparing the materials for Cadus, I worked closely with Larry Hoffman, who Joe had hired as CFO for Cytogen less than a year before I joined. Larry was previously in the same role at The Liposome Company, which was acquired by Elan Corporation plc in May 2000 and was a big winner in my biotech newsletter.

In June 2001, Joe, Larry, and I traveled together to New York City to meet with Carl and Russell to make a pitch regarding AxCell. Joe drove his black Audi and Larry sat in the passenger's seat reading the *Wall Street Journal* during the commute. I sat quietly in the back seat, being the more junior of the trio.

Upon arrival at Carl Icahn's workplace, we were escorted through the opulent offices furnished in mahogany to a meeting room adorned in fine artwork and furniture. In a short while, Russell entered the room. The three of us exchanged pleasantries until Carl made his grand entrance.

Along with immense wealth often comes a big personality and fiery temper, and Carl possessed all of those attributes. The meeting lasted mere minutes as the tough guy from a "rough neighborhood in Queens" provided us with his "take it or leave it" offer for a potential business combination involving AxCell and Cadus.

I give Joe a lot of credit for attempting to negotiate with Carl, but it was quite clear who had the leverage in the meeting—and it wasn't Cytogen. When it became apparent that Joe wasn't going to accept his ultimatum, Carl abruptly left the room. The meeting was over.

We never heard from Cadus again, but the company announced via a press release later that year that it had licensed its yeast-based drug discovery technology to a major pharmaceutical company for an upfront fee of $500,000 and an additional $1 million milestone payment.

Sadly, a few months later, Cytogen mourned the passing of Leslie Misrock—considered one of the longest survivors of prostate cancer.

Shortly before my arrival at Cytogen, Larry had entered into an equity line of credit with Acqua Wellington North

American Equities Fund, Ltd. While equity lines of credit had become quite common, their dubious history landed them the unflattering moniker of "toxic financings." As a result, one of my initial goals at Cytogen was to convince Larry to dismantle the equity facility with Acqua Wellington.

John Nelson, portfolio manager for small-company stocks for the State of Wisconsin Investment Board, one of Cytogen's largest holders, was also quite skeptical of equity lines of credit and sent a warning letter to all the companies in his funds. John was even quoted in an article by reporter Andrew Pollack of *The New York Times* stating, "equity lines of credit might be merely the latest incarnation of toxic financing."

By June 2001, I worked out a deal whereby Cytogen sold 1.8 million shares of stock to the State of Wisconsin Investment Board for an aggregate purchase price of $8.2 million, or $4 ½ per share. In connection with this financing, Cytogen agreed to discontinue the use of the equity financing facility with Acqua Wellington. My mission was accomplished, much to Larry's dismay.

Despite our differing views regarding equity lines of credit, however, Larry was very helpful in guiding us to explore buying a home where he resided in Bucks County, Pennsylvania as opposed to looking in New Jersey. In fact, he took Lorie and me on a driving tour of Yardley that greatly influenced our decision to relocate there. When our house in

Skokie, Illinois sold towards the end of August, Larry also provided us with a referral to Lee Rubin, a local realtor.

It was Labor Day weekend 2001 when we took a trip to Pennsylvania with the goal of buying a new home. Rosie stayed back in Chicago with a friend, but Megan was still nursing and came along. We flew into town that Saturday morning, picked up a rental car, and drove to meet Linda Gallas, who worked with Lee and took us around to see various houses within the parameters we had discussed.

The first house we saw was one that I had found online. From the Internet photographs, it looked perfect. However, upon arrival, we saw a massive water tower directly across the street from the backyard. The interior was also run down and needed a fair amount of work.

After seeing all the houses on our list, Lorie and I were frustrated. We each had picked a different home that would be OK if we had to choose one, but neither of them was what we had in mind. Driving away from the last appointment, we passed a gorgeous house less than a block away with a "for sale" sign out front.

"What about that one?" Lorie asked Linda, who was chauffeuring us around.

"That one's above the price range you gave us," she replied.

"Could we stop and take a look anyway? Just to have something to compare?"

The homeowners were out of town for a few days, but Linda made some calls on her mobile phone and got the combination for the home's lockbox. We pulled into the driveway, and I offered to stay in the backseat of the car with Megan, who was fast asleep in her car carrier.

Linda and Lorie walked up to the front door and disappeared for quite some time. Afterward, Linda emerged from the house alone and walked back to the car shaking her head. I rolled the car window down.

"You're in trouble," she informed me with a smile.

"How's that I asked?"

"Lorie loved the house and said if you're dragging her across the country, this is where she wants to live."

"Oh boy," I exclaimed.

I released Megan from her seat, and the three of us joined Lorie inside. The house was indeed beautiful, and the current owners were downsizing after their kids had grown. There were various items left behind, such as a pool table and couches, which Linda informed us could be purchased with the home or not.

After completing our tour of the house and yard, we decided to place a bid. Lee Rubin had informed us in advance that the local real estate market was quite hot, with most homes selling for full price or even more. We had been pre-approved for a mortgage and made an offer.

Before heading to the airport the next morning, we stopped by to see the house again. As we walked around the backyard we met Roger Yackel, one of the immediate neighbors. He was doing yard work and came over to the wooden fence to say a very friendly hello. He and his wife Sue had just moved in a short while before us.

We returned home to the Midwest. A few days later there was a voicemail message on the machine from Lee Rubin letting us know that the sellers accepted our bid on the house.

———————

Early in the morning on September 11th, 2001, I drove to NYC to attend the Wall Street Analyst Forum investor conference on behalf of Cytogen with my investor relations colleague, Mary Coleman. At the time, I was still commuting by plane from Illinois to New Jersey.

Driving my rental car from Cytogen's headquarters in New Jersey to NYC, we approached the Lincoln Tunnel, which went under the Hudson River to mid-town Manhattan. Mary suddenly jerked her head around on the passenger side.

"Michael," she cried. "Look at that."

She pointed towards the smoke pouring from the top of one of the World Trade Towers, which I could also see as we came around the bend towards the toll booth. Immediately we turned on the car radio to learn more about the situation.

I phoned Lorie back at home with an update in case she saw anything on the news, as I knew she would worry.

"Hey honey, just wanted to let you know that something is going on at the World Trade Center. There's a bunch of smoke emanating from the top of one of the towers. But that is in lower Manhattan and our meeting is in Midtown, so I didn't want you to worry."

"Thanks for letting me know. What do you think is going on?" Lorie replied sounding concerned.

"There's nothing on the radio yet, but perhaps an office fire or gas explosion."

After I hung up the phone and we made it through the tunnel, radio reports started to come in about a small plane hitting one of the towers.

"How the heck does a pilot run into a skyscraper?" I turned and asked Mary. The situation seemed very suspicious.

Just then, reports of a second plane hitting the other tower came over the radio. By this time, I knew something was terribly wrong and attempted to turn the car around and head immediately back to Princeton, but the tunnels were already closed as a precaution.

We had no choice but to drive to our destination at the Roosevelt Hotel on 45th street and Madison. I parked the rental car in the hotel's garage, and we took the elevator to the hotel's lobby. We were only there for a short while watching the news reports on the televisions in the bar area when we witnessed the two towers imploding and crashing into the ground.

For reasons that weren't exactly clear, the venerable old landmark would shortly evacuate. Alarms rang, and people exited the building like cockroaches scurrying out of the kitchen when you turn on the light.

In the confusion and mass exodus from the hotel, I lost sight of Mary and panicked.

"Mary! Mary!" I yelled against the constant sea of people streaming past me through the hotel's revolving doors. But there was no sight of her.

Suddenly, I caught her out of the corner of my eye and grabbed her hand. We ran in the general direction of everyone else, still unsure of what we were even running from.

After a few blocks, Mary and I stopped running and walked around aimlessly, not sure what was happening or where to go. We saw buses pass by, full of people covered in white ashes holding on to the railings while appearing completely emotionless. The entire time sirens from police, fire, and ambulance vehicles roared in the background along with the roar of fighter jets up above.

It was nearly impossible to get a cellular signal and phone anyone. We managed to get a call through to Cytogen and let them know that Mary and I were okay but unsure of when or how we would be leaving Manhattan. We instructed them to phone our spouses and let them know that we were safe in case we weren't able to make any further calls.

Hours passed without further incident, so we went back to the hotel to see if we could retrieve the rental car. Entering the parking garage, we both stopped dead in our tracks as we approached the automobile. The previously empty parking spot next to the car was now occupied by a vehicle that was severely damaged and covered in ashes. It must have been smashed when the towers fell, but how or why it was here now defied imagination.

Setting aside the ominous wreck, we got into our car and headed out. We drove around the city aimlessly for hours, trying to find a way off the island. By early evening, we were one of the first cars across the George Washington Bridge and safely drove back to Cytogen's parking lot for Mary to get her car.

Driving on the New Jersey Turnpike, we realized just how lucky we were. The wind direction blew the thick smoke from the towers away from Midtown. Otherwise, we would have been engulfed in clouds of dust and debris as we wandered the city. Instead, the plumes stretched for miles in a Southerly direction—seeming to follow us along the horizon for a good portion of the ride home.

We kept the radio on for a short while to better understand all that had happened during the day, but after a while, it was too depressing. We drove in silence for the remainder of the trip.

Joe and several others from Cytogen greeted us in the parking lot when we arrived safely back at the office. It was clear that everyone at the office was worried about us all day—mainly since communications were limited.

Arriving at my hotel room in Princeton a short while later, I wept and wept for what I saw that day and all the people who had died, a final tally I didn't yet know. All that I wanted was to be home and hug my family. The next morning, with air travel still grounded, I decided to get in my rental car and drive more than 13 hours straight home to be with my family.

Once more, New York left a bad taste in my mouth. I departed feeling defeated—again.

The shock, grief, and disarray following 9/11 resulted in the purchasers of our Skokie, Illinois home reneging on the deal. Lorie and I loved the Bucks County home and didn't want to lose it, so we decided to take out a bridge loan until the other house was sold. Fortunately, it all worked out, and we moved to Yardley, Pennsylvania in October 2001 to start our brand-new life on the East Coast.

———

At the start of 2002, Joe appointed me as interim CEO for the company's AxCell Biosciences subsidiary with an immediate focus on developing a viable business plan and accessing capital. Cytogen was continually struggling to allocate scarce resources among too many projects, and it became clear that a dedicated effort was needed to focus on AxCell.

Although it was a wholly-owned subsidiary, AxCell operated as a separate entity in Newtown, Pennsylvania, which was less than a 10-minute drive from our home. As such, I set up an office there to oversee the group, which until that time had been handled by John Rodwell, Ph.D., AxCell's president and chief technology officer. As a non-scientist, I was disliked and viewed as an outsider; someone sent in from "corporate" to keep an eye on AxCell.

After developing the business plan, Joe suggested that AxCell engage investment banking firm Ferghana Partners Inc. to assist the company with strategic transactions and corporate partnering. The firm seemed like a good fit since John Rodwell knew one of the members of Ferghana's team, Christoph Pittius, Ph.D. In parallel with Ferghana's efforts, John and I sought commercial partners to utilize the proteomics data that AxCell had generated to date.

On May 9th, 2002, I received an unsolicited email from an executive recruiter looking to fill the president and CEO position for Locus Discovery Inc. in suburban Philadelphia,

Pennsylvania. Locus was a privately-held computational drug discovery company founded in 1999 and was based on technology exclusively licensed from Sarnoff Corporation. The company had 75 employees and $70 million in cash. For the same reasons that I couldn't join Cephalon, I quickly discarded the email without even giving it a second thought.

By September 2002, Cytogen had $16 million in cash and its stock price was below $1 per share. To conserve money, the difficult decision was made to layoff 19 employees at AxCell even as we continued to explore strategic alternatives for the unit with Ferghana. AxCell cost Cytogen about $1 million per quarter to operate—or about one-third of the company's burn rate. The science was promising, but revenue and profitability were far off. As acting CEO, I was charged with delivering the disappointing news to a group of 19 individuals, knowing the negative impact it could have on each of their lives. It was horrible and a reminder that with great power comes great responsibility.

One month later, Cytogen entered into a five-year agreement with Matritech Inc. to be the sole distributor for Matritech's NMP22 BladderChek® device to urologists and oncologists in the United States. Coincidentally, Steve Chubb, who was Cytogen's first CEO, was the founder, chairman, and CEO of Matritech at the time.

NMP22 BladderChek was a point-of-care, antibody-based diagnostic test for bladder cancer that required only a few drops of a patient's urine. The device returned results in thirty minutes and was designed to provide urologists with an adjunct technology to cystoscopy, a clinical procedure for the visual identification of tumors in the bladder.

Similar to the issues surrounding the original merger proposal with Advanced Magnetics, I had expressed concerns about Cytogen licensing NMP22 BladderChek. From a competitive perspective, following the acquisition of Vysis, Abbott Laboratories was marketing Vysis' UroVysion, the first FDA-approved genomic DNA-probe test for identifying early recurrence of bladder cancer. Besides, BTA TRAK®, a competing and potentially equivocal product to BladderChek, was only selling approximately $600,000 per year at $12 per unit, which begged the question of why NMP22 BladderChek was going to be a more substantial market opportunity. More importantly from a strategic perspective, Cytogen continued to bill itself as a therapeutic company, and NMP22 BladderChek was a diagnostic tool.

Nonetheless, during November 2002, Cytogen began promoting NMP22 BladderChek to urologists in the United States using its specialized oncology sales force. Under Joe's leadership, Cytogen was moving into a new commercial growth phase, punctuated by the most comprehensive new product launch cycle in the company's history with the recent introductions of BrachySeed Iodine-125, BrachySeed

Palladium-103, NMP22 BladderChek and hopefully Combidex in the near future.

———

As predicted by meteorologists, a major snowstorm affected the region on Thursday, December 5th, 2002. It appeared that my morning commute from Bucks County, Pennsylvania to Cytogen's headquarters in Princeton, New Jersey could be quite treacherous. However, I felt obligated to make an attempt knowing that the company's chairman, Jim Grigsby, would be at the office starting around 9:30 am to begin an important day of budgeting discussions with senior management for the following fiscal year.

The roads were terrible, but I made it to the office where the parking lot was relatively empty. Most people were delayed coming in, but I was always an early riser and among the first to arrive.

I entered my office, shaking off the snow from my shoes when I was shocked to find Jim sitting at my desk reading a newspaper.

"Come on in, have a seat. It's going to be an interesting day," he said as I stood in the doorway with my jacket and briefcase still in hand.

"What's going on?" I asked extremely puzzled as I sat down in one of the empty office chairs.

"Joe will be resigning from the company, and the board of directors has unanimously supported his strong recommendation to name you as his replacement. We've got a lot of ground to cover, and of course, this is all highly confidential until everything is formalized at the upcoming board meeting. However, I'm sure you'll want to take a moment and call your wife and share the good news, so I'll leave you to it while I grab a coffee, but make it quick."

Still reeling from the news, I phoned Lorie to tell her what transpired and that she couldn't say anything to anyone until the announcement was public.

"You constantly amaze me," she said excitedly on the phone.

"I can't wait to see you tonight and tell you more!"

After spending a fair amount of time meeting with Jim, I walked into Joe's office where he was seated at his desk.

"Well, I certainly didn't see that one coming," I said entering the room and closing the door behind me.

"Yes, I imagine it came as quite a shock. To be sure, the board took some convincing, but in the end, I made a compelling case for you, and they unanimously agreed."

"I don't know what to say, Joe. Other than, of course, thank you for the confidence and support."

"So, do you have a date in mind when you'd like me moved out of 'your' new office?"

I must have looked too much like a kid in a candy store, as Joe replied solely based on my facial cues.

"Ahh, I see. Immediately. Okay then, no problem."

"Tell me, which company lured you away from Cytogen?"

"I need to keep it confidential for now, but I'll fill you in as soon as possible."

At the next meeting on December 17th, 2002, Cytogen's board of directors accepted Joe's resignation as president and CEO, effective immediately, although he continued to serve as a director of the company in full support of the management transition. The board unanimously elected me to the position of president and CEO and also appointed me to the company's board of directors. In connection with these changes, Cytogen's board of directors also accepted the resignation of Larry Hoffman, who left the company to pursue other opportunities.

In the accompanying press release that day, Joe was quoted.

"As we look ahead to the next phase in Cytogen's evolution, I believe it is appropriate that Michael take on an expanded role as CEO. I knew when I helped recruit him that Michael was an outstanding businessman with a very solid grounding in science and technology, and everything he has done since then validates that judgment. With strong support from the senior management team, Michael has identified new business development opportunities and initiated the analysis needed to help make Cytogen a more efficient operating company. Additionally, he has successfully led an intensified focus on presenting Cytogen's business model to our stockholders and customers. I look forward to continued involvement with both Michael and the company as a member of the board of directors."

So, there it was. At age 34, I had just been given the proverbial keys to the Cytogen kingdom.

In her typical supportive fashion, my stepmother Linda emailed me soon after the press release went out: "So now, what have you wanted to accomplish with this company...it is within your grasp. Set your sites and go for it—you will achieve it."

Less than a week following Cytogen's board meeting and officially being appointed CEO, I felt the need to celebrate. After work one day, I decided to drive to a Porsche-Audi automobile dealership in Conshohocken, Pennsylvania to lease a new car. Something younger, sportier—more fit for a CEO to drive, as opposed to my silver Mercury Grand Marquis, a full-size, rear-wheel-drive luxury sedan associated with a much older demographic. I ended up leasing a $40,000 green pearl 2003 Audi A6 with a beige leather interior.

Lorie laughed at my shameless self-celebration but took a victory lap or two around the block with me.

"Have to admit," she smiled, "it's a pretty cool car."

Apparently, I wasn't the only person to receive that unsolicited email from an executive recruiter back in May 2002 looking to fill the president and CEO position for Locus Discovery Inc. On January 6th, 2003, it was announced that Joe Reiser had been appointed to the job.

Taking a quick inventory of the company I had just inherited; the situation was rather bleak. Cytogen had less than $15 million in cash at the end of 2002, which would barely last a year. Total revenue had only increased 10 percent from the prior year, which was below analyst and investor expectations. Quadramet, the company's flagship therapeutic product heralded as a billion-dollar opportunity, was still struggling to grow in the hands of commercial partner Berlex. And, by implementing a reverse stock split, Cytogen had just narrowly escaped having its stock delisted from trading on the prestigious Nasdaq exchange and moving to the Pink Sheets. At the end of December 2002, Cytogen's market valuation was a mere $31 million—a far cry from $1.5 billion just a few years prior. I felt like I had just been handed the keys to the Titanic after it hit the iceberg and was charged with getting all of the passengers and crew safely to shore.

I knew that I could accomplish anything I put my mind towards and certainly wasn't going to give up. So, I started restructuring Cytogen's product portfolio away from lower margin, higher volume products, and diagnostics. Cytogen sent Draximage notice of termination concerning the BrachySeed products in January 2003. By that time, it had become clear that the brachytherapy market was commoditized and Cytogen was in no position to compete solely on pricing.

Fortunately, Cytogen received some good news that same month with the announcement of a research collaboration between AxCell Biosciences and biotech industry bellwether Celgene Corporation to research specific ubiquitin ligases and their role in cancer and inflammation. Ubiquitin ligase targets were of great interest to several large pharmaceutical companies, including Merck and Johnson & Johnson, which helped validate the importance of the field. Unfortunately, while the industry recognized the potential of these drug targets, the early leads failed to demonstrate efficacy. Still, interest in the ligase targets remains, and one day this drug class might represent a breakthrough for treating cancer and other diseases.

Next were back-to-back financings, where Cytogen sold shares of newly issued common stock and warrants to institutional investors seeking to build a decent position in the company. The first $5 million was raised in June at $4 ¾ per share and then $10 million raised in July 2003 at $8.53 per share. The fact that Cytogen was raising money even as its stock continued to rise was a strong signal that investors believed in our business model and supported our proposed use of capital. The financings allowed Cytogen to buy back the marketing rights to Quadramet in North and Latin America from Berlex Laboratories. Under the agreement, Cytogen agreed to pay $8 million upfront to Berlex and royalties based on future sales.

I felt that the reacquisition of marketing rights to Quadramet provided an excellent opportunity to accelerate Cytogen's product-driven, therapy-focused business model, which was viewed favorably by our investors. In addition to providing pain relief, emerging data indicated that Quadramet could potentially be used in combination with other drugs, such as chemotherapeutics and bisphosphonates, to treat a variety of cancers.

Next, I began building out the senior management team, including the promotion of Bill Goeckeler as senior vice president of operations in January 2003, Chris Schnittker as CFO in September 2003, Tom Lytle as senior vice president of sales and marketing in April 2004, Bill Thomas as senior vice president and general counsel in August of 2004, and Dr. Mike Manyak as vice president of medical affairs in December 2004.

In November 2003, Cytogen completed a registered deal resulting in gross proceeds over $20 million at a price of $11 per share. In a registered direct offering, the company files a shelf registration statement with the SEC in advance of the anticipated need for funding, which allows the registered shares to be taken "off the shelf" when market conditions are ideal. Because investors receive fully liquid, registered securities, they are not in a position to demand onerous terms or discounts, so such financings are generally more efficient and less costly to the issuer.

The financing was used primarily to double the company's commercial infrastructure from 25 to more than 60 individuals along with other investments in the sales, marketing, and clinical development of the company's products.

In April 2004, Cytogen raised another $26 million through a registered deal priced at $10.10 per share. That year, the company's revenue derived from product sales reached a record $14.6 million. Cytogen was also added to the Russell 3000 Index, which comprised the 3,000 largest U.S. stocks. Institutional ownership in the company grew threefold.

In recognition of all these accomplishments, I was nominated and became a finalist for the Ernst & Young Entrepreneur of the Year (EOY) award in both 2004 and 2005.

———

Twenty-five years is a long time in the life cycle of any company, especially in biotechnology where discoveries can change entire fields seemingly overnight. For two and a half decades, Cytogen had put itself on the biotechnology map with leading science and had invested nearly $400 million researching and developing new products since inception. Going forward, however, I expected the company to be best known for commercializing exciting new oncology products— one of which I hoped would be Combidex.

In early March 2005, senior management from both Advanced Magnetics, Inc. and Cytogen Corporation traveled to Gaithersburg, Maryland to jointly participate in the FDA's Oncologic Drugs Advisory Committee (ODAC) meeting to review the regulatory filing for the Advanced Magnetics product Combidex, and ultimately decide the investigational product's fate.

In September 2004, Advanced Magnetics had submitted a complete response to an approvable letter the company received from the FDA back in June 2000. At the time, an approvable letter was one of 3 outcomes from the FDA review process, other than "approved" and "not approvable." It can mean that the FDA wants more data, wants label revisions, wants some post-marketing studies or has other questions.

Combidex was being positioned to help physicians distinguish between cancerous and non-cancerous lymph nodes in patients with primary cancer at risk for lymph node involvement. For instance, if prostate cancer is lymph node positive, surgical removal of the prostate gland may be rendered unnecessary, and in bladder cancer, the risk of death increases by 20 percent with each additional positive lymph node.

In the absence of Combidex, the only noninvasive way to assess lymph nodes was with various imaging techniques that merely relied on measuring the physical size of the lymph node. In general, lymph nodes smaller than one centimeter are considered benign, while lymph nodes greater than one centimeter suggest the presence of cancer. But size alone is insufficient for an accurate diagnosis, and a technique that detects and characterizes lymph nodes with a high degree of sensitivity and specificity is needed.

Combidex is comprised of tiny small particles of iron that are injected into the bloodstream and are subsequently taken up by a specific cell called a macrophage that is found in healthy but not malignant lymph nodes. Twenty-four hours later, during an MRI procedure, normal lymph nodes turn black due to the uptake of iron in macrophages, while cancerous ones remain white on the resulting image because they don't contain iron. Thus, the images produced using Combidex could be used to help guide biopsy or image-guided dissection for improved staging.

Following a publication of independent study results in the prestigious *New England Journal of Medicine*, Combidex had generated significant interest from the medical community. However, when the FDA asked members of the

ODAC committee if they thought that the data demonstrate that Combidex was safe and effective for marketing approval based on Advanced Magnetics' proposed indication, the vote was overwhelmingly negative: 15 to 4.

Everyone was in shock.

The hopes for Combidex were extremely high before the ODAC committee meeting. Analysts covering Cytogen's stock projected $100-200 million in revenue and the company's sales force was eagerly awaiting an exciting, new product to market to their customers.

We stayed in our preparation room at the hotel in Gaithersburg, Maryland to finalize the disappointing press release that would go out that afternoon. We also spoke with numerous investors that called our cell phones trying to understand what had just happened.

It didn't matter that Combidex was Advanced Magnetics' product and we were ostensibly the marketing partner. Both companies took a hit on the negative outcome. Advanced Magnetics' stock nosedived 65.1 percent to close at $6.65, while shares in Cytogen plunged 51.9 percent to $6.26 on the day of the announcement. Shares of Cytogen never fully recovered from the setback and didn't trade in the double-digits ever again.

Following the meeting, Advanced Magnetics received a second approvable letter from the FDA with certain conditions. Cytogen would later file a breach of contract lawsuit against Advanced Magnetics seeking damages along with a request for specific performance requiring Advanced Magnetics to take all reasonable steps to secure FDA approval of Combidex in compliance with the terms of the licensing agreement. The suit would ultimately be settled, with Advanced Magnetics paying $4 million to Cytogen and releasing shares of Cytogen common stock being held in escrow. In addition, both parties agreed to early termination of the 10-year license and marketing agreement and supply agreement established in August 2000. Ultimately, the conditions of the second approvable letter were never satisfied, and as a result, Combidex wasn't approved by the FDA.

As someone who generally prefers to be in control, I didn't like the fact that Cytogen had no jurisdiction over the product's development. I was frustrated that our company shared the blame for the ODAC meeting outcome and that we had no near-term product candidate to fill the void created by the rejection of Combidex.

I received numerous phone calls and emails from Cytogen's sales reps asking nervously what the company planned to do next in the wake of Combidex. There was hope that the product could have been approved and launched in 2005 and our sales reps were struggling to grow our legacy radiopharmaceutical products. I knew we needed to license a new product or technology soon, and that it must be a marketed or soon-to-be-marketed product or our sales force would start seeking jobs elsewhere. But to do so, we first needed to raise money.

For several years, I had been interacting with local venture capitalist Jay Moorin of ProQuest Investments, a healthcare-focused venture capital firm founded in 1998. Jay is a seasoned healthcare executive whose background includes senior roles in leading investment banking, pharmaceutical, and biotech companies.

By June 2005, it appeared that we were getting closer to having ProQuest invest in Cytogen. I wrote to Jay in early June 2005.

"As always, I really enjoyed our meeting on Friday. I truly hope we can find a way to connect ProQuest and Cytogen in the coming days or weeks."

"We discussed Cytogen with our partners yesterday and they agreed with our recommendation to take a quick and hard look at making a major investment. Obviously, we have followed your progress over the past few years and think you are one of the better CEO's we know," Jay wrote back to me.

On July 19th, 2005, Cytogen announced it was raising $14 million through the sale of 3.1 million shares of registered common stock priced at $4.50 per share and 776,000 warrants to purchase shares with an exercise price of $6 per share to ProQuest Investments and OrbiMed. No investment banker was used in this transaction.

Jay emailed me after the transaction.

"I did this deal because I trust you. If I ever lose that feeling, we'll sell your stock in a nanosecond."

Beyond the much-needed cash, Jay's introductions to key members of the prostate cancer community were invaluable. Through Cytogen's joint venture with Progenics, we were already close with key opinion leaders at MSKCC like Howard Scher, M.D. and Susan Slovin, M.D. But now Cytogen was invited to the prestigious Prostate Cancer Foundation scientific retreat in September 2005, where we got to meet other essential contacts.

Chapter Six
Dear John

———

Lorie and I made several family trips during 2005 with Rosie and Megan, including Puerto Rico for the Fourth of July weekend and a trip to the Hamptons in late August. But I felt like I needed to clear my mind of the recent stress from the FDA's decision not to approve Combidex and revisit hiking for the first time since my 1998 family trip to Canada.

"Lorie," I said after dinner one night, "I'd like to take a little trip off by myself."

"What for?" she asked.

"I just need to clear my head and decompress. This Combidex non-approval mess has thrown me for a loop. Cytogen can't seem to catch a break—it's almost like the company is cursed."

"OK," Lorie said. "I get it, and agree you definitely deserve a break."

"Thanks for understanding. I hope it works."

I decided to book a hotel room for a few days near the southern terminus of the Delaware Water Gap National Recreational Area in Pennsylvania. This 70,000-acre watershed atop the Pocono Plateau stretches for forty miles on both the Pennsylvania and New Jersey sides of the Delaware River. It's about a 2-hour drive from our house, and I mapped out several exciting day-hikes in the area.

As I was also starting to explore photography more seriously, I packed my new Sony Cybershot DSC-F828 camera, arguably the best digital camera priced between a professional and consumer level. What futurist Alvin Toffler called a "prosumer" product that had been released the prior year. The decision to bring my camera would spark a fledgling hobby in photography in years to come.

I set out on my first hike on Monday, August 29th, 2005, from the Dingmans Falls Visitors Center parking lot. The 5-mile trail began on a wooden walkway that took me to the foot of Silver Thread Falls, where water from a tributary to Dingmans Creek drops 80 feet through a narrow shale crevasse, cascading over a series of ledges. The walkway continued to a viewing platform, which is the end of the tour for non-hikers. I continued the hike with a short climb into the forest on a well-worn, root-covered trail that mostly followed the creek-side through a hemlock ravine. The trek concluded with three uniquely different waterfalls: Deer Leap, Fulmer, and Factory. There's also a stone ruin, a reminder that the waters from Dingmans Creek have run several mills throughout the years.

For Tuesday's hike, I went up Mount Minsi, another 5-mile loop starting from the parking lot for Lake Lenape. The hike started at the trailhead for the Appalachian Trail and just a mere half-mile into the walk, I could see the cars and 18-wheeler trucks whizzing along Interstate 80. But at this altitude, I didn't have to hear any of the traffic noise, and each time I stopped for a view, the trucks and cars got smaller as I climbed higher up the rocky cliff edge of Mount Minsi. After reaching the peak, I looped back to the Appalachian Trail and continued until I reached Sunfish Pond, which was covered in blooming lily pads and the occasional frog.

It was raining on Wednesday, so I decided not to hike and just spent the day relaxing. During my drive back to the hotel the prior day, I'd seen a billboard advertising that American rock band ZZ Top was performing a show at the Mountain Laurel Center Wednesday night. I had my laptop at the hotel, so I went online to search for tickets. Surprisingly, there were still some available for purchase. Even though I went alone, it was a small venue and one of the best concert performances I've attended.

I left the hotel on Thursday, September 1st, 2005 to drive several hours to my last day-hike at Ricketts Glen State Park, home to a series of wild, free-flowing waterfalls, each cascading through rock-strewn clefts in an ancient hillside. The 94-foot Ganoga Falls is the highest of 22 named waterfalls. Old growth timber and diverse wildlife added to the beauty of the hike.

I was all smiles when I got home that night. The walks alone in the woods had served me well.

"Guess the time-out worked," Lorie said. "At least for now."

———

Hiking in the Delaware Water Gap National Recreational Area only fueled my interest in being more adventurous, but I didn't want to do it alone. Fortunately, John Tedesco, Cytogen's senior director of quality and operations, was much more of an outdoorsman and had even published a book on nymph fishing, a specialized form of fly-fishing.

Our families first met years ago at a work-related party for Cytogen. John's wife Maureen taught elementary school, like Lorie. John had reassured her that this party would be different from the usual biotechnology techno-talk crowd since one of his coworkers also had a wife who was an elementary school teacher.

John introduced Lorie and me to his family as soon as we arrived.

"Lorie and Michael, I'd like you to meet my wife Maureen and daughter Kaitlyn."

"Nice to meet you both," we replied in unison.

Kaitlyn was around eight years old and the apple of her daddy's eye. You wouldn't know it at all by looking at her, but she suffered from a rare disease called spina bifida, a tethered spinal cord. Most of her young life had been spent in hospitals, wheelchairs, and operating rooms. Ultimately, she would have over 25 surgeries to repair, or untether, her spinal cord. Her case was rare, as many people who have spina bifida as bad as Kaitlyn don't walk or breathe on their own. She'd been in pain most of her life, with little relief, but was always upbeat, energetic, and happy.

"Hello Mike and Lorie," Maureen responded.

"Michael doesn't go by Mike, Maureen, so make sure you call him Michael," I overheard John whisper in her ear.

Rolling her eyes, I'm sure Maureen thought I was just another stuffed shirt that she wouldn't be able to talk to that evening.

As the night progressed, however, Maureen enjoyed several hours of conversation with Lorie and getting to know her and all about our girls, who weren't there on this occasion.

Maureen also talked about their two older sons, John and Brian, and all about education. It was the beginning of a beautiful friendship between our families.

"John and I have been married almost 25 years," Maureen told Lorie. He's changed jobs eight times."

"Wow," Lorie exclaimed. "That must have been tough."

"Definitely," Maureen agreed. "John is no social butterfly, but with your husband, I noticed a huge change. He talks about Michael like they were brothers. Michael's younger, but he has the same type of drive as John and many of the same interests. John says they can talk for hours, something I've never seen before in my husband's personal life."

While Lorie and Maureen were having this discussion, I was busy telling John about my recent hiking adventure and seeing ZZ Top, which he wouldn't believe until I showed him the ticket stub I kept in my wallet.

"What do you think about hiking the AT," John asked out of the blue.

The Appalachian National Scenic Trail, generally known as the Appalachian Trail or AT is the longest hiking-only footpath in the world, ranging from Maine to Georgia.

"Sure," I said. "That's a great idea, but we don't have the time to do the whole thing at once."

An Appalachian Trail thru-hike takes between five and seven months to complete the entire trail.

"That's OK," John went on. "We can hike it in sections. A little bit each year until we finish the whole 2,190 miles. Let's start at the Delaware Water Gap."

"Excellent solution. As your boss, I approve the time off," I kidded him, "and also take it for myself."

The Delaware Water Gap National Recreation Area is home to 28 miles of the Appalachian Trail, which was a logical starting point for our journey. We targeted the Kittatinny Ridge, which towers over a thousand feet above the Delaware River, offering rich views of the area.

At first, I was quite apprehensive about spending a long time trapped in the wilderness with a colleague. I don't do well with the small talk bullshit. What if he babbled incessantly during the hike? It was a very unusual situation for me to place myself in, but we began planning our walk in early October, with plans to leave on Friday, October 21st, 2005 and return Sunday, October 23rd, 2005.

Not being much of an outdoorsman, I had to purchase a lot of supplies for the extended trip, including a tent, backpack, cooking gear and more. I also read about encounters with black bears along the trail, so I purchased what I assumed to be a decent sized knife for protection.

"John, come take a look at my computer screen," I said proudly one afternoon when he came to my office. "I want to show you the knife I ordered online for our hike."

"For what purpose?" he asked.

"Protection. You know, from black bears."

John studied the screen for a moment and then smirked. "That's nice. Hopefully, it will give me a solid running start while you're busy pissing off the bear poking him with that thing."

Clearly, John knew a lot more than I did about serious camping.

On Friday, we drove separately to the northern location where we expected to end the hike and left my car parked there. Next, we traveled together to the southern starting point for our 24-mile journey and parked John's car there. Adding to my apprehension about the trip was the fact that there was no turning back once we started—our only viable option was to hike until we reached my car.

My backpack was quite heavy, weighing about 70 pounds when I set it on our bathroom scale back home. It contained 2 gallons of water, a tent, sleeping bag, clothing, and food. It was difficult to stand, let alone walk with it on my back.

We started out in the morning and reached our first objective by dinnertime. A good portion of the first section was uphill, and I was exhausted as we set up camp for the night.

The clearing we found had the remains of a fire pit, so we set up our tents and started a fire. To pack lightly, John and I stocked up on dehydrated food—the stuff that turns into a hot meal when you add boiling water. We sat on a fallen tree trunk in front of the fire, eating our hot meals and enjoying the serene setting.

"You know what, after hiking all day this food tastes pretty good," I said somewhat surprised.

"I have to agree, in fact, I'm going to bring some home for Kaitlyn to try," John replied.

After we finished eating, it started to get dark even though the night was young.

"I hate to say it, John, but I'm beat. I think I'm going to go crash for the night," I informed John as we packed up the cooking gear and hoisted our backpacks way above ground using parachute cord to avoid attracting bears or other animals.

"Sure, no problem. I'm going to stay up a while and enjoy the fire, but you go ahead."

Before I made a move, amid the peace and calm— *BANG!* Our entire campsite was briefly lit up as if a flashbulb had gone off. John and I were stunned as seconds later a large, full-antlered deer bolted crookedly through the campsite. Clearly injured, it disappeared quickly into the darkness beyond the trail.

"Hope I didn't scare you fellas," a burly man carrying a big double-barreled shotgun entered into our campsite. "Did you happen to see which way the deer went?"

My ears were still ringing from the gunshot, and I hadn't fully grasped what had just taken place, but I managed to point in the direction the deer ran without saying a word.

"Much obliged," he said, continuing in pursuit of his game.

Meanwhile, John ran right after the hunter.

"Be right back," he hollered to me as he scampered off.

He came back a few minutes later, somewhat out of breath.

"What the hell?!" I said.

"I knew that deer was done for and dropping soon right nearby," he explained. "So, I wanted to make sure our friend, the big killer, didn't leave any parts behind that could attract bears or any other animals you're always so worried about."

"Holy cow," I said, still rendered motionless.

"I know, at first I thought we were being shot at," John replied. "Go on to bed. Hopefully, that's all the excitement we'll have tonight."

Despite the adrenaline rush, I fell asleep in my tent within seconds. I had nothing left; every ounce of energy was drained from my aching body. Peace returned to the campsite. Only the occasional cracking and snapping from the fire broke the silence.

My deep slumber was interrupted a short while later by the sounds of children talking and laughing. At first, I thought I must have been dreaming—until I heard John's voice.

"Keep it down, please," John said to the boy scout leader and his troop. "My boss is in the tent over there asleep."

"Oh gosh," the scout leader replied. "We were hoping to set up camp here. It's dark, and the kids are getting tired."

"Nope," John said authoritatively. "There's another campsite up a bit farther. You'll have to make it there for the night."

That was John, always looking out for me. Beneath his Grizzly-Adams, tough-guy exterior was a warm and gentle man who was loyal to those close to him. He wasn't going to let a group of kids disturb my sleep; not on his watch. A small, kind and selfless gesture that further cemented the trust and respect I had for him.

I quickly fell back asleep or more precisely passed out from sheer exhaustion.

———

Waking up the next morning, I was pleasantly surprised what a difference a good night's sleep had made. I wasn't sore and felt refreshed. The campfire had gone out, so I went without my morning coffee instead of starting it back up again.

I yelled to John through his tent, and he emerged shortly after that. We lowered our backpacks from the trees and headed back out on the trail. The temperature dropped overnight and a dense layer of morning fog blanketed the campsite.

After hiking for a few hours, we came across a clearing. Echoing from beyond the field was a strange sound, almost like an animal in pain or distress. Not seeing anything, we continued.

"John...John!" I yelled at him. "Look!"

I pointed beyond the field where we saw a mother bear and two cubs. They were a reasonable distance away, but not far enough for my taste. Everything I read regarding bears said to avoid a mother and her cubs, as they are very protective of their young. Immediately, I had visions of the bear charging at us.

Don't worry; you've got that knife to protect us, I envisioned John mocking me.

John and I stood still, allowing greater distance between the bears and us as they continued to march along. Moments later we heard the same wounded animal sound, as a lone cub ran to catch-up to the rest of its group. Soon, the mother bear and all three of her cubs moved out of the field and disappeared deep into the forest.

By afternoon, the heavy rain started. John and I were prepared, so we donned our rain gear and pushed forward. The forest canopy provided periodic protection from the rain, but the wet rocks of the Appalachian Trail in that area were treacherous to walk. One slip could result in a twisted ankle or worse.

Over the last 40 miles or so of the AT in Pennsylvania heading north toward New Jersey there are only two shelters— structures with an overhanging roof, a wooden floor and three walls, also known as a "lean-to," available for thru-hikers. Fortunately, we stumbled upon the Kirkridge Shelter, which is the last shelter for northbound hikers in Pennsylvania. It was built in 1948, and the accommodation was weathered and worn but had a dry wooden floor that could sleep up to eight people. The rain-soaked ground was too wet for pitching our tents, so we decided to end that day's hike and spend the night in the Kirkridge Shelter.

The temperature dropped to 35 degrees Fahrenheit that night. With an open wall and cold temperatures, it was much harder to sleep than previous nights. Making it even more difficult was the fact that John snored. Badly, in fact. I didn't realize it when we were in separate tents spaced apart, but his gurgling and rough rattling noise echoed loudly against the walls of the shelter.

The next morning, the final day of our hike, we were greeted by a spectacular sunrise peeking through the trees, as the opening of the lean-to faced towards the east. Sitting on the open edge of the lean-to, I brewed a pot of coffee and watched the sun glistening through the beautiful autumn leaves, which were covered in droplets of rainwater.

By mid-day, we reached Mount Minsi and stopped to take some photographs as we neared the end of our adventure. After taking individual photos, I put the camera on timer mode and snapped a picture of the two of us. Rather than looking tired and frazzled from the trip, our expressions captured the pride of completing the first of our many planned excursions.

After packing up my car, we stopped at a nearby fast-food drive-through on our way to get John's car at the other end of our trip. We were ravenous, and the warm meal never tasted so good.

When I finally arrived home, Lorie greeted me as the garage door opened.

"Wow, you are disgusting!" She exclaimed, halting her hug in mid-embrace. "Take your clothes off now and go directly to the shower."

"OK. Yeah, I bet I'm pretty ripe," I replied, "...haven't bathed since I left and just hiked more than 24 miles."

Once I was in the hot shower, I reflected on the hike as the dirt and grime built up during the past several days circled the drain. What amazed me most about the trip was that even though neither of us made friends easily, John and I got along extremely well. I don't usually know how to be anything other than intense. I'm always searching, always questioning, always trying to find the meaning in everything. I think of myself as sometimes too passionate and stuck in my head, and as a result, am sometimes misunderstood. But John was okay with all that, and I looked forward to our next adventure.

———

They say that money doesn't buy happiness, but it does let you rent it. My position at Cytogen allowed us to spoil our girls with vacations and much more. For example, Rosie was infatuated by dolphins as a youth, so we booked a trip to Florida in November 2005 so she could experience swimming and interacting with them at Sea World.

We enjoyed the Victorian elegance and modern sophistication at Walt Disney's lavish Grand Floridian Resort, which let us visit the various theme parks or enjoy spending time at the pool.

Rosie was quite comfortable in the water and even used a snorkel and goggles to swim around. Being a few years younger, Megan was still a bit apprehensive about putting her head entirely underwater. Accordingly, she wore pink eye goggles and an inflatable Ariel-themed jacket over what she adorably called her "bathing woot."

"Watch me dive, Daddy," she said while wearing a floatation device.

"How are you going to dive? You don't like going underwater," I replied laughing.

"I'm going to be an above-water diver," she replied matter-of-factly.

Almost from the moment she was born, Megan was a happy child. She had an infectious smile and laugh. It was rare for her to pout or be angry for any length of time.

Unfortunately, the morning we were all scheduled to go to Sea World, Megan got the stomach flu, and Lorie offered to stay back with her at the hotel so that Rosie didn't miss her dolphin adventure.

When Rosie and I arrived, we were escorted to a changing area where we put on wetsuits and were prepped for the day's agenda. I'm not sure who was more excited about swimming with the dolphins, Rosie or me.

Entering the water, the animal trainer brought one of the dolphins over to Rosie to pose for a photo. The trainer gave Rosie instructions on how to support the dolphin's lower jaw with both hands cupped as she kissed the animal on the nose.

Snap! Went the Sea World photographer's camera.

Next, we waded out away from the shoreline to a staging area where trainers would get two dolphins to bring us back to shore by holding on to their fins.

We were carefully positioned in a spot where we could grasp the dolphin's fins.

"Hold on, tight, you guys," the trainers yelled at us, smiling. "Just let the dolphins do the work!"

Then...WOW!... We suddenly sped off like a shot, the water streaming behind us as if we were water skiers hooked on a speedboat, cutting through the spray and foam...ten...twenty...fifty yards until we saw the shore again and heard the trainers shouting.

"Let go...you can stand up now!"

Which we did, breathless with joy and excitement.

Back at the hotel later that evening, Lorie and I enjoyed some quiet time together after the kids fell asleep. I briefed her on the dolphin adventure, although I felt bad that she and Megan had missed out.

"I wish you were there to see how excited Rosie was to be among the dolphins," I said to Lorie before sipping a glass of red wine as the two us were lying in bed.

"Me too, but I'm glad you were able to go with her," Lorie said. "I can tell that you had just as much fun as she did, you big kid."

"We'll have to get the picture of her kissing the dolphin blown up extra-large and hang it in her room."

"Aw, I think she'd love that."

While work at Cytogen could be stressful, it was times like this that made it all worthwhile. Lorie believes Walt Disney is indeed the happiest place on earth, and for that moment in time, it indeed was for all of us.

———

For reasons I'll never fully understand, John had kept a rather large secret from me. In April of that year, John had been diagnosed with osteosarcoma after finding a lump on his left leg. Having a portion of his leg removed, plus several lobes of his left lung and a round of radiation, the last thing he should have done was go hiking with me on the AT.

Maureen was anything but thrilled at the thought of John going hiking, but never revealed his secret. At the time, she seemed more upset that we were taking the trip during her birthday weekend, which I thought was a bit of an overreaction at the time. However, I later came to appreciate how she felt in her heart that it could be her last birthday with John. I felt horrible afterward.

It was so surprising. John was in front of me the entire time during our hike and never showed any signs of being tired or in pain. In fact, he was in a lot of pain and taking medication the entire time, including when he ran off spontaneously after that crazy hunter with the double-barreled shotgun. Maybe he was worried how his diagnosis would affect his job? Or perhaps just afraid of being treated differently.

After coming clean about his diagnosis, John was adamant about continuing to do stretches of the Appalachian Trail each year—just as we had initially planned.

"I'm doing more than a mile every day on the treadmill, so I should be ready for one of those 'easy' hiking sections this spring!!" he emailed me optimistically one day.

For the Holidays that December 2005, John got me the book *A Walk in the Woods* by Bill Bryson. Inscribed inside the front cover, he wrote: "Michael, looking forward to doing more of the AT with you!! Happy Holidays!! John"

Maureen later confided to Lorie that as their lives began to change forever, John instructed her to ask me if she ever needed anything.

"He's a good man, Maureen," he told her.

"What makes Michael so different from anyone else you have worked with over the past 25 years?" she asked.

"He's decent, wants to do what is right and knows what the fuck he is talking about. He is not a bull shitter. I would trust him with my life."

Among our similar interests was our taste in music. In connection with his 60th birthday, Pink Floyd band member David Gilmour released *On an Island*, his third solo album, in March 2006. Being huge fans, John and I had each purchased the album. Hearing it for the first time in our respective offices, we compared notes via email.

"Listen to the title track – awesome," I wrote John.

"Excellent – I like the guitar on the first track as well!! Actually, can't wait to get in the car and turn this up!"

The next day, I again wrote to John.

"I just watched the video to the cover track from Gilmour's new album on his website. I don't know about you, but I recall a much younger David Gilmour when I last saw Pink Floyd in concert. It makes me feel ancient as well!"

"Well, he is getting older," John replied, "but remember – we hiked nearly 25 miles or so on the Appalachian Trail, so we're also doing okay for a couple of old guys. "But hey," he went on, "I'd love to see him live in concert. I'm definitely in if he does!"

Knowing John's cancer diagnosis, I wanted to do something special for him. Sure enough, Gilmour made a tour stop at the Rosemont Theatre in Rosemont, Illinois. I tried to get two tickets through my American Express Platinum concierge service, but the agent set low expectations as many of his shows sold out quickly.

As it turned out, fortune smiled upon us.

"I've got some good news and some bad news," I said to John two days later in my office at Cytogen.

"Start with the bad news, boss."

"All three Gilmour shows (New York, Illinois, California) are sold out."

"*Great*. And the good news?"

"You and I have tickets for the show on Wednesday, April 12th, 2006 at the Rosemont Theatre, just off center stage."

"No way!! That's incredible. How did you pull it off? Also, let me know what I owe you," John said enthusiastically.

"The fine folks at American Express have a concierge service for Platinum Card members, and they were able to score the tickets. Don't worry about the cost, though; they're on me. You can buy the beer that night."

A few weeks later, John and I met in Chicago the day of the concert. I booked dinner reservations at Smith & Wollensky's chophouse right on the Chicago River. We had quite a meal and decided to walk around town for a bit before the show to burn off some calories.

Later that evening, John and I saw David Gilmour play live. It was an amazing performance, with Gilmour covering his entire new solo album along with a lot of songs from Pink Floyd—including *Wish You Were Here*. I was happy for the experience but more pleased that John was there and got to see Gilmour live—perhaps for the last time. I think John smiled throughout the entire show.

Inspired by heartbreak over the self-imposed exile of Pink Floyd's founding guitarist and first leader, Syd Barrett, I listed to Gilmour sing a familiar phrase.

"How I wish, how I wish you were here."

I knew when, or more optimistically "if" John were to pass that we were trying to squeeze years of experiences and memories into what was likely going to be a concise time. And I knew at that moment that the song *Wish You Were Here* would hold much deeper meaning to me at some point in the future.

———

I continued efforts to turnaround Cytogen, including the sale of the company's 50 percent interest in its joint venture with Progenics later that month for $13 million upfront and potential future milestone payments totaling up to $52 million and royalties on product sales, if any. As a commercially-focused company, we allotted almost all of our budget to sales and marketing activities as opposed to research and development, and the joint venture only diluted Cytogen's scarce financial resources. More importantly, the product candidates being developed through the joint venture were taking longer than initially expected, so the divestiture made sense.

To help improve the company's margins, Cytogen also entered into a royalty buyout agreement with Berlex, Inc. for Quadramet. Under the terms of the agreement, Cytogen would no longer pay Berlex a royalty on Quadramet sales in exchange for a one-time cash payment of $6 million, future sales-based milestones, and the issuance of 623,441 shares of Cytogen common stock to Berlex.

Cytogen's primary products, Quadramet and ProstaScint, were both radiopharmaceuticals, which had historically been a challenge to market—not just for Cytogen, but even for much larger pharmaceutical companies like GlaxoSmithKline plc that struggled to market Bexxar® (tositumomab combined with iodine 131). Accordingly, I knew what Cytogen needed was to acquire non-radiopharmaceutical products or technologies following the FDA's rejection of Combidex. To accelerate this process, we engaged ProPharma International Partners in April 2006 as an extension of our internal business development outreach to see if they could uncover any assets that we might have missed. ProPharma's role was to identify, analyze, and negotiate product or pipeline opportunities for Cytogen.

In parallel, we continued to explore therapeutic product leads from other sources. One such prospect arose from a research collaboration with James Gulley, M.D., Ph.D., who was director of the clinical immunotherapy group at the National Institutes of Health (NIH).

I first met Dr. Gulley while attending the ASCO annual meeting in the summer of 2005. He had expressed an interest in conducting clinical studies combining Cytogen's Quadramet product with an experimental therapeutic vaccine for prostate cancer, as he believed there could be synergy between the two approaches.

It had taken some time for him to wrap-up the necessary preclinical studies, but by March 2006 we met again at the American Association for Cancer Research (AACR) annual meeting where a poster with some of his preclinical data was being presented.

Shortly after that, Dr. Gulley submitted the Quadramet study to the NIH's Scientific Review Committee. One of the items that arose during the review was covering the high cost of Quadramet. With budget cuts, the NIH was naturally looking for ways to conserve money.

Because Quadramet was a radiopharmaceutical product and subject to rapid decay, the drug couldn't be stored, and new batches had to be manufactured on a weekly basis. Further, since the company didn't know the exact demand for the drug each week, we produced slightly more drug than needed so that we never had to turn down a prescription. I informed Dr. Gulley that we had extra product available for him and would be happy to supply free Quadramet for the study, for which he was quite grateful.

In early August 2006, Dr. Gulley mentioned Therion Biologics based in Cambridge, Massachusetts during a telephone conversation. Dr. Gulley and others at NIH had developed an "off-the-shelf" cancer vaccine platform, which Therion was testing for both pancreatic and prostate cancer. It was the same prostate cancer vaccine Dr. Gulley was exploring in his Quadramet combination study.

The following month, Cytogen initiated discussions with Therion and its investment bank to assess whether or not there was synergy between the two companies. Unfortunately, interest in Therion Biologics wasn't supported by our research and development team. To be fair, there was a lot of skepticism about cancer vaccines and immunotherapy approaches following some high-profile failures at the time.

Ultimately, the call was mine as CEO. However, if I had approached Cytogen's board of directors to do a strategic deal that didn't have the blessing of our R&D team, I would be taking a huge and potentially fatal risk. We passed on the opportunity.

Following the failure of its lead vaccine candidate in pancreatic cancer, Therion filed Chapter 7 in November 2006. The technology reverted to the NIH and would later be licensed by Danish biotechnology company Bavarian Nordic, which initially focused solely on advancing the prostate cancer vaccine. In the coming years, Bavarian Nordic advanced the prostate cancer vaccine to Phase III development and landed a partnership with pharmaceutical giant Johnson & Johnson. Bavarian Nordic saw its market cap climb substantially as a result.

Regardless of whether or not Bavarian Nordic's prostate cancer vaccine ultimately succeeded in the clinic, I believe passing on Therion was a mistake. It could have been strategic for Cytogen, especially by bolstering the company's presence in the prostate cancer community.

———

Since September is prostate cancer awareness month, Cytogen developed a marketing campaign titled "Screen, Stage and Support" that was initially launched in September 2001. The initiative was designed to help men learn about the importance of early screening and detection, proper staging and diagnosis, and the many support resources available for people living with prostate cancer—one of the most common types of cancer affecting men.

An essential element to the "Screen, Stage, and Support" initiative was arranging for Cytogen to ring the open bell at Nasdaq each year during the first week of September in honor of prostate cancer awareness month and to highlight the three central components of the Screen, Stage, and Support program. Knowing that many of the popular financial media outlets, such as CNBC and Bloomberg, covered the Nasdaq openings, I believed that we could get added media exposure for our events due to the unique prostate cancer message. For added insurance, however, we would enlist the help of celebrities to give added visibility. Such stars included NY Yankee baseball legends Yogi Bera (2001 & 2002), Whitey Ford (2003), and Lou Piniella (2004).

Cytogen's fifth and final "Screen, Stage, and Support" event was one of my personal favorites. On September 1st, 2006, former New York City Mayor and prostate cancer survivor Rudy Giuliani joined with Cytogen to help kick off prostate cancer awareness month by ringing the Nasdaq Stock Market's opening bell. Also, leaders from the American Cancer Society, the American Urological Association, Michael Milken's Prostate Cancer Foundation, and Us TOO International also joined together at the market open to formally launch Cytogen's annual Screen, Stage and Support campaign.

Cytogen put out a press release quoting Giuliani to announce the event.

"Recognizing that proper screening and diagnosis can save your life is key to being a prostate cancer survivor. That is why Cytogen's 'Screen, Stage and Support' campaign is so important. Together, we can help more men and their families get a proper diagnosis and the treatment and help they need to beat prostate cancer."

Gathering at the Nasdaq MarketSite that morning, there was energy in the air as stock ticker symbols and quotes scrolled across the sizable electronic wall behind the stage where we would all soon gather. Photographers worked the room, taking pictures of Rudy with various event participants. As one of the more high-profile events Cytogen had ever done, Lorie and our daughters were there in support and to enjoy a few minutes of television fame as the Nasdaq openings were broadcast live across most of the financial outlets.

Lorie had dressed Rosie and Megan in matching dresses for the event. Everyone, including them, wore a blue-ribbon pin symbolizing prostate cancer awareness along with an elastic blue bracelet with Cytogen's logo and the words "prostate cancer awareness" embossed in white.

More than 30 individuals, including board members, employees, and various prostate cancer organizations took the stage at Nasdaq's MarketSite moments before the 9:30 am Eastern Time opening bell to receive instructions on where to look, how long to clap, and how to exit the stage. To ensure that they weren't lost among the group of adults, the Nasdaq organizers thoughtfully positioned Rosie and Megan right in front of the podium. They were the stars of the show.

Giuliani, Lorie, and I were positioned behind the podium, but I could see our little girls buzzing together with excitement on the bright LCD screens mounted around the room reflecting the live footage.

3...2...1

The stage came to life with applause as Rudy and I rang the opening bell. As instructed, Rosie and Megan stood to clap in front of the podium, grinning from ear-to-ear for all to see across the nation.

As hoped, CNBC interviewed Rudy and me immediately following the opening bell ceremony. There I was, seated next to Rudy Giuliani, doing a live television interview about prostate cancer awareness and Cytogen.

Dad and Linda watched the CNBC segment back in Chicago and phoned later to congratulate me.

"We couldn't be prouder of you and your family," said my father.

"Thanks, Dad. It means a lot to me for you to say that. It was a bit nerve-wracking, but I thought it went well."

"You handled yourself very well, and Rudy gave good credit to Cytogen."

"Yeah, I was a bit disappointed that the interview veered off topic a bit from the prostate cancer message, but overall it was a spectacular success."

"Lorie coordinated her dress with what the kids were wearing perfectly. Very fitting for the wife of a CEO. We understand that a television producer is ready to offer big bucks for future media rights to include Rosie and Megan."

"Ha! They were adorable standing there clapping during the opening ceremony! We got some great pictures that I'll send you."

In addition to the Screen, Stage and Support campaign, Lorie and the kids joined me each year for another prostate cancer event. Cytogen helped support the local New Jersey chapter for the American Cancer Society's "Run for Dad" program held each Father's Day. Many of Cytogen's employees would participate in the 5K run, including me, which helped build comradery. It was a carnival-like atmosphere, with face-painting and other activities for the kids.

———

Through the business development efforts of ProPharma International Partners, a unique product opportunity was identified called Caphosol®. We moved quickly to license the exclusive North American rights from a Norwegian family-owned company called InPharma AS.

Caphosol, a topical, oral agent, is a prescription medical device. It's an adjunct to standard oral care in treating oral mucositis caused by radiation or high-dose chemotherapy, a condition estimated to affect more than 400,000 cancer patients each year. Caphosol is also indicated for dryness of the mouth (hyposalivation) or dryness of the throat (xerostomia) regardless of the cause or whether the conditions are temporary or permanent.

During our due diligence process, I learned quite a bit about oral mucositis—an inflammation of mucous membranes in the mouth with symptoms ranging from redness to severe ulcerations. Virtually *all* patients receiving radiation therapy to the head and neck areas develop oral mucositis and approximately 40 percent of patients who receive chemotherapy develop some form of oral mucositis during their treatment. Also, more than 70 percent of patients undergoing conditioning therapy for bone marrow transplantation develop oral mucositis.

On October 11th, 2006, Cytogen announced that it had licensed North American rights to Caphosol from InPharma in exchange for an upfront fee of $5 million upon the closing of the transaction and an additional $1 million payment after six months. In addition, InPharma would receive royalties and sales-based milestone payments. The deal also provided Cytogen with the option to acquire the rights to Caphosol for the European and Asian markets.

The next day, Asbjorn Hanson of InPharma visited Cytogen's office. We had interacted via phone and email throughout the negotiations, but this was our first time meeting in person. Holding a box of Caphosol, the two of us posed for a photograph in front of Cytogen's corporate logo in the office lobby to memorialize the event.

Caphosol works by lubricating the mucosa and helps maintain the integrity of the oral cavity through its mineralizing potential. The distinguishing feature of Caphosol is its high concentrations of calcium and phosphate ions, which are hypothesized to exert their beneficial effects by diffusing into intracellular spaces in the epithelium and permeating the mucosal lesion in mucositis. Calcium ions play a crucial role in several aspects of the inflammatory process, the blood clotting cascade, and tissue repair and phosphate ions may be a valuable supplemental source of phosphates for damaged mucosal surfaces.

A prospective, randomized, double-blind, placebo-controlled trial demonstrated Caphosol to be a significant adjunct in the management of mucositis associated with high-dose chemotherapy and radiation therapy. The trial evaluated 95 patients undergoing hematopoietic stem cell transplantation with the duration and severity of mucositis and requirements for opioid medications prospectively assessed. Data demonstrated significant decreases in days of mucositis, duration of pain, dose of morphine, and days of morphine use for patients receiving Caphosol as compared to those administered a placebo.

By the time of Caphosol's acquisition, in addition to my formal title of CEO, I was managing both finance and sales due to turnover in each of those departments. It was a lot to take on and, in retrospect, too much. A fact that didn't go unnoticed by Jay Moorin at ProQuest, who addressed his reply to my email sharing the good news about Caphosol with "Dear Michael Becker, CEO, CFO, VP Sales" and the phrase "get some help." It was clear that Jay's patience with Cytogen's inability to grow the radiopharmaceutical business was dwindling and reading between the lines, I knew that if Caphosol didn't start off strong, we were likely to lose his trust and support.

Looking back, ProPharma International Partners first identified InPharma in March; seven months later the licensing deal was done. The average time from introduction to close for most deals ProPharma had found was 9 to 12 months. I was proud that our team acted so quickly and thoroughly to bring the project to closure.

As his disease progressed, John Tedesco had both radiation and chemotherapy treatment. But keeping busy was very important to John—his work meant a lot to him, and he took great pride in it. So, I let him start working from home over the summer of 2006.

In almost every email to me, he kept referencing going on our next hiking trip. He was in denial about his disease virtually from day one, but by autumn he finally started facing reality. His wife, Maureen, would email me updates on his condition and mental status. Sometimes John would phone work and colleagues told me that he wouldn't make any sense. Other times, he insisted on having Maureen drive him to Cytogen so that he could return to work, but we always managed to find excuses to keep him home.

In September 2006, we had our last joint family dinner at the Cheesecake Factory near King of Prussia, Pennsylvania. It was a happy occasion, with Kaitlyn, Rosie, and Megan goofing around while the adults made small talk.

By October, John's condition declined rapidly. Disoriented, he would send odd emails about his disease being stable and plans to start driving again soon. His very last email to me was on October 25th, 2006—almost exactly a year after our hiking trip. It was short and sweet—congratulating me on the hiring of a Kevin Bratton as Cytogen's new CFO. Shortly after that, hospice was called in.

On October 28th, 2006, the final Saturday of the month, I visited John for the last time at his house. Lorie and Maureen took Kaitlyn out shopping so John and I could have some time alone. Somehow, I think John and I both realized it would be the last time we'd see each other.

John passed on November 4th, 2006. Memorial and funeral services were held several days later near John's home. Maureen asked me to say a few words during the memorial, for which I was honored.

After my remarks, I joined Maureen and her three children who were commenting that it was a good day for fishing since it was raining and perhaps a sign from John for everyone to keep moving forward. As they described, rain was good for fishing because the light rain makes casting lines more discreet. Also, insects are more likely to be out flying near the surface of the water during or immediately following a light rain, which will bring fish closer to the surface and make them more susceptible to being caught.

After discussing the weather and fishing, I had a chance to speak privately with John's youngest son, Brian, who was 24 years old at the time.

"You know, your dad and I were planning to hike a portion of the Appalachian Trail each year until we finished it," I said solemnly to Brian. "I'll never forget the beauty of the last sunrise we saw from the Kirkridge Shelter after a night of rain. You see some magnificent sights while hiking."

"Yeah, I have seen hundreds of Alpine sunrises, all magnificent, but none as awe-inspiring as the sunrise on August 2, 1990, when we were living in Colorado," Brian replied. "It was my eighth birthday, and of course, Pops and I were hiking. At eight years old, I was already checking Colorado 'fourteeners' off my list. In just two years, Pops and I had checked off 15, which isn't too bad given the short, two-month summer climbing season. Unfortunately, our family would soon move to San Diego, ending the goal of summiting all fourteeners."

In the mountaineering parlance of the Western United States, a fourteener is a mountain peak with an elevation of at least 14,000 feet.[8] In Colorado, there are 53 fourteeners with at least 300 feet of topographic prominence.

"I imagine you get a pretty good view of the stars from that high altitude and it must be quite peaceful up there," I replied.

"There are few things more marvelous than watching the sunrise while sitting at the base of The Diamond, the sheer and prominent east face of Longs Peak. It is a world-famous Alpine climb. Being above tree line, at approximately 13,000 feet, the massive granite face rises to over 14,200 above and the sky is magnificent. The Milky Way is brighter than anything seen at lower elevations, the stars almost seem within reach, and there is no distraction between you and the beauty of the heavens. As the sun rises and the black darkness of night gives way to the pink hues of morning, the stars of the Milky Way fade to give way to the sun."

After John's passing, Maureen and their oldest son John moved to Ohio where he graduated from Case Western Reserve University, while Brian and Kaitlyn moved back to Colorado. Despite the distance, we still keep in touch. Kaitlyn is currently in school at the University of Colorado Boulder. Brian's desire to finish conquering all of the fourteeners kicked in; even if it's now just him completing that goal.

At every summit, Brian places a picture with his dad under a rock—the highest rock. The reason being, and for anyone who knew John this would make sense, if you are going to climb a mountain, you need to stand on the highest rock; otherwise, what's the point?

Last I checked with him, Brian also inherited his father's love for fishing and had been sidetracked with spending summer days on the South Platte. But the goal continues, and the photo of Brian with his dad now sits buried at the top of 28 fourteeners.

"Each summit attained is accompanied by a few tears, laughs, and reflection, but most importantly, each summit is accompanied by appreciation," Brian later told me. "Appreciation of lessons learned and experiences had. I will, at some point, stand on top of the +50 highest summits in

Colorado and fulfill our dream—most likely accompanied by a few tears—and while he will not be with me in person, he will be with me in spirit and the lessons he taught me."

"Everyone has their happy place," Brian continued. "Mine is in the Rocky Mountains of Colorado, whether hiking Alpine trails or fishing in the half-light of a canyon stream, where so many memories I wish I could relive are stored and held on to and kept safe, no matter how much time passes. While life takes the things we want to hold on to most dearly before we are truly ready to let go, life also leaves us lessons and memories that can shape our perspective. For me, that beauty is sitting on a rock in August 1990 at 13,000 feet, having breakfast with my dad. It's a beauty I can't replicate, but also a beauty I can carry with me, which I do every day."

Chapter Seven
The Great Recession

———

It was tough to go back to work after losing John, especially during the winter months. This time of year is usually difficult for me due to seasonal affective disorder (SAD), also known as the winter blues. As the days grow shorter and light becomes scarce, SAD is a type of major depression that emerges and affects an estimated 10 million Americans. While the exact cause isn't known, the reduction in sunlight during winter may reduce levels of Vitamin D and serotonin (a brain chemical that regulates your mood) and increase levels of melatonin (a chemical which regulates sleep and mood).

Typically, my attitude improves during the spring months with increasing daylight. However, May of 2007 turned out to be an exception. Izzy Englander, who ranked among the ten most famous hedge fund managers at the time, filed a 13D with the Securities and Exchange Commission (SEC) reflecting his newly acquired 1.7 million shares, or 6 percent stake in Cytogen. Millennium Management fund became the third largest holder of the company. In contrast to 13G filings that indicate a passive investment, a 13D filing suggests a non-passive investment or potential activist role.

The purchase of a large number of shares in a company often results in upward price movement, but Cytogen's shares were largely unaffected. The lack of price movement leads me to believe that Millennium had negotiated a cross transaction with another fund that already owned Cytogen shares and was looking to sell. I figured the seller was likely ProQuest Investments, which last reported a 6.4 percent stake in Cytogen. A future SEC filing would confirm ProQuest eliminated its entire position in Cytogen.

We had recently met with Millennium to introduce the fund to Cytogen as we regularly did with prospective investors and there was no indication that Millennium had any activist intent. Further, Millennium had filed 13D's for several other biotech companies in the prior month—including a 6.3 percent stake in ArQule Inc., a 5.2 percent stake in HearUSA Inc., a 7.2 percent stake in Orchid Cellmark Inc., and a 7.1 percent stake in VistaCare Inc.

In a fairly standard disclosure, Millennium said in each of the 13D filings that from time to time they might hold discussions with third parties or with management concerning potential changes in the operations, management or capital structure of such companies as a means of enhancing shareholder value. Talks could include such matters as disposing of or selling all or a portion of the company or acquiring another company or business, changing operating or marketing strategies, adopting or not adopting certain types of anti-takeover measures and restructuring the issuer's capitalization or dividend policy. Millennium stated in the filings that the firm did not have any present plans or proposals that relate to or would result in any of the actions mentioned above.

Coincidentally, the very next day, Bill Kridel of Ferghana Partners left me a cryptic phone message stating that he would like to discuss a European company that happened to be in NYC but said it was nothing that he could put in an email. I suspect the European company must have been EUSA Pharma based on subsequent events.

Around this time, Cytogen was making plans to raise additional capital to support the commercial launch of Caphosol. We also started exploring other investment banking relationships beyond Rodman & Renshaw and decided also to include Roth Capital Partners LLC. Companies generally receive more favorable financing terms by selling freely tradable, registered shares and we expected to utilize that approach. Unfortunately, a covenant from the previous financing in late 2006 precluded Cytogen from selling shares at a price less than $4 per share for six-months, or until June 28th, 2007. The company's stock had been trading around $2, so there was no opportunity to utilize the company's registered shelf. Further, in early June we learned that the company's shelf had gone "stale" due to the decline in market capitalization. All of this meant that we couldn't utilize the shelf and would have to do a financing using unregistered shares, which usually came at a much higher cost to the issuer.

We were hoping to do a larger financing with sophisticated biotech investors who would take a longer-term view of Cytogen and its investment prospects. In this regard, we met with Bay City Capital, Caxton, and several others capable of doing a single, large transaction. However, when it became clear that accessing registered shares for a financing was not an option, we shifted gears to do a smaller raise until a new registration statement became effective.

On June 4th, 2007, I received an unsolicited fax from EUSA Pharma, which had initially expressed an interest in European marketing rights to Caphosol. The letter was complimentary of Cytogen's progress and pipeline, and Bryan Morton, president and CEO of EUSA, stated in the letter that "We have carefully studied the Cytogen business through publicly available information, and industry sources, and based upon what we have learnt, we would like to explore a potential combination of our businesses through an all-cash offer for the outstanding shares of Cytogen."

After discussing the development with Cytogen's board members and legal counsel, I responded to Bryan's letter stating that Cytogen was not interested in pursuing a transaction of that nature. However, if EUSA would like to continue discussions on the possible licensing of Caphosol in Europe, I let him know that Cytogen would be happy to do so after execution of a mutually acceptable standstill agreement, a contract that stalls or stops the process of a hostile takeover. I was confident in our business and future, as Cytogen had just announced new sales and marketing leadership with the appointment of Stephen Ross as senior vice president of sales and marketing.

———

The financial crisis of 2007–2008 is considered by many economists to have been the worst financial crisis since the Great Depression of the 1930s. The active phase of the crisis, which manifested as a liquidity crisis, can be dated from August 9th, 2007, when BNP Paribas terminated withdrawals from three hedge funds citing a "complete evaporation of liquidity."

While not the more substantial transaction Cytogen had envisioned, against this economic backdrop we were fortunate to conclude a $10 million private placement financing on June 29th, 2007, by selling 5.8 million common shares at a price of $1.74 per share with 2.9 million warrants priced at $2.23 per share. Introduced by Rodman & Renshaw, Brian Pinsker of JP Morgan participated in the deal. During our initial discussion, he had proposed that Brigette Roberts of Third Point Partners, a noted activist investor, also join our meeting for which we politely declined—especially given the recent 13D filing by Millennium Management. Sensing blood in the water, the sharks were circling.

Not surprisingly, Brian Pinsker became somewhat of an activist himself and began sending me emails. At first, they were relatively benign notes, such as "after earnings you should consider buying stock in the open market as I think that is the best sign for investors." Then they graduated to warnings, like "Not sure why your selling, general, and administrative costs are so high. You will need to raise money in 3 months at this rate. I don't want to be diluted below my cost." Finally, Brian requested to speak directly with Cytogen's chairman, James Grigsby.

At this point, I handed the communication to our general counsel who contacted Brian via email to determine the nature of the call and types of questions being asked. Brian responded quickly.

"Ok, I guess given I am the largest shareholder of CYTO, and the stock is down 60 percent in the past three months, and I have never listened to or spoke directly to the chairman I thought it would be worthwhile to introduce myself and to listen to his vision. Anyway, the conversation is meant to be more of an introduction that's all."

The call was scheduled for October 2007, and I didn't need to hear from Jim after the discussion. I instinctively knew that Brian viewed me as a roadblock to consummating a strategic transaction and was likely looking to get me out of the company.

Due to growing concern for shareholder activism by Izzy Englander or Brian Pinsker, combined with a deteriorating general business climate and the overall difficulty of biotechnology companies in obtaining financing, Cytogen explored the pros and cons of retaining an investment banker to assist the company with investigating various strategic alternatives, including the possible sale of Cytogen.

To this end, in November 2007, the board of directors retained ThinkEquity as its investment bank to evaluate potential strategic alternatives available to Cytogen to enhance the future growth of Cytogen's pipeline and maximize stockholder value. I knew investment banker Ken Moch from our time together at the Biotechnology Council of New Jersey (BCNJ) where he served as chairman, so ThinkEquity seemed like a good fit. After the press release went out, Brian Pinsker sent me an email stating that he was very pleased Cytogen was trying to maximize shareholder value.

Cytogen's product sales were $15 million for the nine months ended September 30th, 2007 and for the first time the company was on track to total more than $20 million in sales for the year. Caphosol had been introduced in March 2007 and revenues for the third quarter of 2007 were $409,000, reflecting a 75 percent increase over the amount reported in the second quarter of 2007.

I received an email from Linda Chisholm, an executive recruiter with CEO Resources, on October 1st, 2007, stating that her firm was performing a confidential retained search for the CEO of a development stage, oncology-focused biotech company in the Mid-Atlantic region.

Intrigued, especially since Cytogen could potentially be sold, I offered to send her my resume and expressed interest in learning more. We exchanged phone calls and emails during the week and set up a meeting for Monday afternoon with Linda Resnick, the head of CEO Resources. She was planning to attend a panel discussion where I was speaking at the Biotech 2007 conference, an annual joint symposium by the

BCNJ and Pennsylvania Bio. Held in Philadelphia, Pennsylvania, we agreed to meet during the event.

My panel session was titled "Invention vs. Acquisition: Strategies for Successful Pipeline Growth" with other panelists including Daniel Greenleaf, CEO of VioQuest Pharmaceuticals, Jane Hollingsworth, CEO of NuPathe and Matthew Gantz, CEO of Acureon Pharma. I was seated next to Dan, who had recently joined BCNJ, and we made small talk before the start of the session. Earlier that year, BCNJ announced during its annual meeting the election of new officers, with myself being appointed the chairman, and three new members to its Board of Trustees, including Dan. We exchanged business cards and planned on keeping in touch following the event.

After the panel, I walked down the short set of stairs to exit the stage and was greeted by Linda Resnick.

"Michael Becker?"

"Yes indeed," I replied.

"Great panel," she said. "It's a pleasure to meet you in person finally. Shall we find a quiet place to sit and talk for a few minutes?"

"Likewise, and yes...let's go find a quiet corner."

After finding a spot, Linda began talking to me in a hushed tone.

"I'm sure you are curious to learn the identity of the confidential company we are representing."

"Yes, you have me in suspense. What is the company?"

"VioQuest Pharmaceuticals."

"VioQuest?" I thought for a brief moment, and then the lightbulbs went off in my head.

"Wait a minute! I just met the CEO of VioQuest," I exclaimed. "We were seated next to each other on the panel. He seems like a nice guy. Boy, this is awkward."

Linda and I discussed VioQuest in greater detail, including its office location in Basking Ridge, New Jersey, which is over an hour drive from Bucks County. More unsettling than the potential commute was the fact that Dr. Lindsay A. Rosenwald and his family beneficially owned 19 percent of VioQuest's outstanding common stock. As a result, Dr. Rosenwald might have the ability to exert significant influence over the company.

Why could that be problematic? Before founding Paramount BioCapital in 1991, Dr. Rosenwald was managing director of corporate finance for D.H. Blair & Co., a privately-owned investment firm headed by J. Morton ("Morty") Davis. D.H. Blair underwrote hundreds of companies, many in the biotechnology industry. The firm was known for investing in biotech companies, pumping their stocks, and then short selling them out of existence. D.H. Blair ceased retail operations in April 1988, and several of its executives and employees were indicted for fraud years later. Rosenwald, however, was not charged.

Beyond any potential concerns about Lindsay's affiliation with VioQuest was the company's poor financial condition. As of September 30th, 2007, VioQuest had a mere $2.5 million in cash and nearly that amount in accounts payable obligations. The company needed to raise more money. Fast.

During my tenure at Cytogen, I secured more than $100 million in new capital for the company. On that basis, I was confident—perhaps *overly* sure—that raising money for VioQuest wouldn't be a problem, especially given the company's diverse oncology pipeline, which consisted of three clinical product candidates.

We negotiated various terms of my employment letter, which included a competitive salary. I was also eligible to receive sizable milestone-based bonuses. The bonuses ranged from $150,000 to $2 million and were based on increases in VioQuest's market value.

After speaking with various board members, Lindsay's office phoned me on October 25th, 2007 to set up a meeting with him at Paramount BioCapital in New York the following day. His luxurious corner office was on the 48th floor of 787 Seventh Avenue. The 45-minute encounter went well, and we discussed some of the open salary and bonus structure issues.

The following week, I sent an email to Steve Rocamboli, VioQuest's chairman, stating that while I considered myself to be quite a rain-maker, "I'm concerned about the length of the runway I will have to secure the needed financing given the company's cash balance and burn rate." I stated that my decision on whether or not to join VioQuest would be significantly enhanced if we could structure some small bridge financing from Paramount or another source to extend the company's runway.

Steve set up a call with Lindsay on Sunday, November 4th, 2007. Lorie, Rosie, Megan and I were eating lunch at the Cheesecake Factory near King of Prussia, Pennsylvania when my cell phone rang.

"Hello?"

"Michael, it's Lindsay."

I stood up and walked away from the table to find a quiet space just outside the restaurant.

"Thanks for taking time on a Sunday to speak with me. I'm quite optimistic about VioQuest's pipeline and future, but there's one concern that is keeping me from accepting the position."

"Yes, what is it?"

"Well, I've been successful at raising money in the past, but as you know the financial markets are a bit shaky at the moment. I'm concerned that I won't be able to raise money quickly and VioQuest only has about six months of cash. Would it be possible for you or Paramount to commit to backstopping any financing need if the market conditions deteriorate further?"

"Of course. I've never let one of my companies go under."

"Excellent, then I think we can move forward on that basis."

In retrospect, tackling an important issue such as a future funding commitment should have been dealt with in a more formal, written manner as opposed to a quick verbal agreement on my cell phone. It is a perfect example of why those of us from the Midwest are correctly stereotyped as being too friendly and trusting.

At a meeting of Cytogen's board of directors in early November 2007, I announced, and the board of directors accepted, my resignation from my executive officer and director positions, effective as of the close of business on November 9th, 2007. At that same meeting, William J. Thomas, Cytogen's then current senior vice president and general counsel, also announced his resignation from his executive officer positions. In response to the departures, the board of directors appointed Kevin G. Lokay, a member of the board, as president and chief executive officer of Cytogen.

Then I had a big surprise.

The board of directors also approved Executive Retention Agreements with each of Cytogen's current executive officers, including Kevin J. Bratton, senior vice president, finance and CFO; William F. Goeckeler, senior vice president, operations; and Stephen A. Ross, senior vice president, sales and marketing; and one of Cytogen's key employees, Thu Dang, vice president, finance.

The retention agreements were infuriating, as both Bill and I had firmly and repeatedly recommended to Cytogen's board of directors that it would be customary and prudent to adopt an employee retention plan for key officers in merger and acquisition situations. Had the board acted on our recommendation, I wouldn't have considered leaving Cytogen at the time.

————

On November 14th, 2007, VioQuest Pharmaceuticals announced my appointment as president, CEO, and director, effective November 21st, 2007.

"The Board of Directors is pleased to welcome Michael Becker as President and Chief Executive Officer of VioQuest. We believe his impressive leadership skills, business development accomplishments, industry expertise, and successful capital raising track record make him the ideal candidate for the job. Further, we have great confidence that Michael's experience leading a company focused on the treatment and supportive care of cancer patients will prove valuable as we work to better leverage our existing asset base and advance new strategic initiatives to accelerate growth and build sustainable value," said Stephen Rocamboli, chairman of VioQuest.

Of the three drug development programs that VioQuest was pursuing, new legislation signed into law September 27th, 2007 made one of them potentially quite valuable.

The FDA Amendments Act of 2007 added a new section whereby a drug developer with a treatment for a neglected disease—diseases that are infectious or parasitic and typically affect large populations in poor developing nations—could receive a "priority-review voucher" from the FDA for the expedited review of a second treatment of the firm's choice.

Priority review vouchers were often described as "Willy Wonka's golden ticket," and could be made available to the highest bidders. Economists at Duke University, who first published on this concept in 2006, estimated that priority review could cut the FDA review process from an average of 18 months down to six months, shortening by as much as a full year the time it takes for the company's drug to reach the market.[9] For a company with a top-selling drug with a net present value close to $3 billion, the Duke researchers calculated the accelerated approval could be worth over $300 million. Under the legislation, the resulting voucher could also be sold or bartered to another company or acquired as part of a buyout of its owner.

To qualify for the vouchers, the drugs or biologicals seeking approval for a neglected disease, often referred to as tropical diseases, must be a new chemical entity. Drugs also must target one of 16 specific conditions to qualify for the vouchers.

VioQuest was developing sodium stibogluconate (SSG) as a selective, small molecule inhibitor of specific protein tyrosine phosphatases, with demonstrated anti-tumor activity against a broad spectrum of cancers both alone and in combination with other approved immune activation agents, including IL-2 and interferons. VioQuest had licensed oncology rights to SSG from the Cleveland Clinic Foundation and was developing the drug as a protein tyrosine phosphatase inhibitor for a range of potential indications.

In addition to its potential role as a cancer therapeutic, however, SSG has been used in many countries around the world as a first-line treatment of leishmaniasis, a protozoan infection typically found in tropic and sub-tropic countries. Historical published data and a large observational study conducted by the U.S. Army, including data from approximately 400 patients, were to support VioQuest's New Drug Application (NDA) with the FDA. The U.S. Army was interested in having SSG formally approved by the FDA for the treatment of leishmaniasis, as opposed to using a non-approved drug on soldiers fighting in the Middle East.

Upon FDA approval, VioQuest could have been among the first companies to receive a priority review voucher. With the company facing financial trouble, the voucher seemed like an excellent asset to potentially leverage for investment.

Knowing my former Cytogen colleague Dr. Mike Manyak maintained an avid interest in field exploration and expedition medicine, and also edited a textbook on expedition medicine, I engaged him as a consultant on the SSG project.

––––––

On March 10th, 2008, I was at my desk at VioQuest when I read the press release that EUSA would merge with and into Cytogen, with the latter becoming a direct, wholly-owned subsidiary of EUSA. At the effective time of the merger, each share of Cytogen's common stock would be canceled and converted automatically into the right to receive $0.62 in cash for an aggregate purchase price equal to $22.43 million.

As of December 31st, 2007, Cytogen had $9 million in cash, but close to that amount in accounts payable and accrued liabilities. As projected, product sales were a record $20.21 million that year. Having watched the company's value previously soar as high as $1.5 billion, it was a sad day. The finality of the news hit me very hard.

By the end of 2007, JP Morgan had increased its Cytogen holdings to 4.6 million shares, or 13 percent. Interestingly, in November 2008, Brian Pinsker, who most recently worked on JP Morgan's healthcare proprietary trading desk, departed the firm to launch a healthcare hedge fund called 11:11 Capital Co. LLC, which was coincidentally seeded with significant capital from Millennium Partners.

No one could have foreseen what would happen next. In September 2008, mortgage giants Fannie Mae and Freddie Mac were taken over by the government, Bank of America agreed to purchase Merrill Lynch for $50 billion, and Lehman Brothers filed for bankruptcy-court protection. On September 29th, 2008 Congress rejected a $700 billion Wall Street financial rescue package, known as the Troubled Asset Relief Program, or TARP, sending the Dow Jones industrial average down 778 points, its single-worst point drop ever.[10]

When I approached Lindsay Rosenwald about an injection of capital to keep VioQuest going, he reneged on our verbal agreement citing the financial crisis. Over the past year, the company had undertaken a broad-based and intensive effort to raise capital, find a strategic partner, or sell the company or its assets. VioQuest was represented in the process by Paramount BioCapital.

Since there were insufficient funds to support the company's continuing operations, I provided written notice to the board of directors of my intent to terminate employment for good reason as defined in my employment contract. VioQuest soon disappeared, as did Paramount BioCapital. In 2009, however, Lindsay Rosenwald and another individual founded a new company called Opus Point Partners. The company specializes in healthcare and life sciences investments and consulting.

What a calamity. After all the ups and downs and changes of the past few years, I was unemployed, out of work, done with all that I'd struggled so very hard to preserve and grow.

Against the backdrop of everything that happened at Cytogen and the subsequent challenges with VioQuest, I entered a dark period in my life. The milestone of having just turned 40, the stress of finding work, and uncertainty in the global financial markets culminated in an existential crisis.

In existentialist philosophy, the term "existential crisis" specifically relates to the moment at which an individual questions if their life has meaning, purpose, or value. For years, I had been caught up in the constant work grind to not only survive, but thrive. And I had accomplished that goal in each of my professional pursuits—computers, finance, and biotechnology. But there had to be more from life than just working a job, paying bills, and ultimately passing away.

Even when things had been going well, traveling for work and the long hours took time away from my family. In some ways, I felt like I was just a paycheck to them. I had accomplished so much—especially from where I started as a teenage screw-up—and yet I was left questioning whether or not my life had any meaning, purpose, or value.

What if my life was cut short, just like John Tedesco's, would I one day be forgotten? John had his fishing book published, but what would I leave behind beyond my family? My mind wandered to religion, and whether or not my decision to convert to Judaism somehow robbed Rosie and Megan of all the cherished memories I had growing up— celebrating Christmas, Easter, etc. Would the absence of such memories make it even easier for them to forget me?

I'm not an overly religious person, but I started questioning my faith and everything around me. The topic of discarding Judaism for my original Lutheran upbringing and introducing issues like putting up a Christmas tree in the house put a significant strain on our marriage. Lorie took the kids to Chicago a few times, and the subject of divorce even circled.

I was a mess and fully expected Lorie to leave me. She had every right. But for some reason, she truly loves me. And it was that love that allowed her to see things through, for which I am eternally grateful.

———

After a great deal of soul-searching following my experiences at both Cytogen and VioQuest, and at the height of the financial crisis, I decided that I needed to form my own business. It would be starting something from scratch, as opposed to trying to "fix" someone else's mistakes like Cytogen and VioQuest. No board of directors, no stockholders to please; the choices would all be mine to make—for better or for worse.

On November 10th, 2008, I officially launched a consulting firm focusing on investor relations and public relations called MD Becker Partners LLC. While the "MD" represented the initials of my first and middle name, I liked the subliminal "doctor" message given the firm's focus on the life sciences sector.

In contrast to all of the prior "talks" with Lorie, the conversation about starting my own business was quite brief. I explained that landing a new CEO position could take up to several years, especially given the financial crisis. Further, the flexibility to work from home could provide more time and access to the kids. In many ways, I thought that starting my own business could help bring us all closer together.

"You know how I hate the uncertainty of what your monthly paycheck will be when you're not receiving a steady salary," she said. "And with everything going on in the financial markets right now, there's an added risk."

"I know, but I don't see many financially stable biotech companies that would be good targets for me as CEO in the current climate. There are a lot of walking-wounded that have only a few months of cash left, and I don't want to step into another mess like that."

Lorie didn't say anything for a while, but I knew she was thinking seriously about what I'd just said.

"OK," she said finally. "If anyone can succeed in investor and public relations it is you, so let's go for it."

After creating a website for MD Becker Partners and other collateral materials, I asked Debbie Hart of BioNJ to provide a brief quote to use in the November 10, 2008 press release announcing my new venture.

"As Chairman, Michael brought BioNJ to a new level when he drove our new brand and proposed the establishment of the annual Dr. Sol J. Barer Award, two impactful moves which provide insight to the creativity, vision, and passion for the industry and region that will drive his success in this new venture."

During my tenure as chairman from 2007-2008, I led a rebranding campaign for the Biotechnology Council of New Jersey (BCNJ). In September 2007, the organization officially became BioNJ. Accompanying the new name was a fresh logo designed by Roessner & Co., which depicted a DNA chain within the outline of the State of New Jersey. The branding reflected the substantial growth of BioNJ since its founding in 1994 to become the only organization in the state solely devoted to the interests of biotechnology-driven enterprises, while more closely aligning BioNJ with the larger, national trade group, the Biotechnology Industry Organization (BIO).

Another one of my goals as chairman was raising the profile of local biotech success stories, such as Celgene Corporation. In this regard, I first proposed the idea of an annual award named after Sol J. Barer, Ph.D., chairman and CEO of Celgene Corporation at the time. Celgene is a New Jersey success story that began with 35 employees in 1998 and a decade later had almost 2,000 dedicated employees in more than 30 countries around the world.

In March 2008, Sol was presented with the first "Dr. Sol J. Barer Award for Vision, Innovation, and Leadership." The annual award recognizes the outstanding research and business leaders who have made and continue to make significant contributions to the growth of the biosciences in New Jersey and around the world. Each year, the honoree is voted on by the BioNJ Board of Trustees from nominations taken from the Nominating Committee.

Due to the financial crisis, there were a lot of unemployed executives starting to do consulting. Most of them were dismissed as "single-shingles"—people with cheap business cards, AOL email addresses, and no vision of growing beyond a one-person shop. In fact, for many of them, it was merely a veiled attempt to land a new job after being out of work.

I wanted to stand out from that crowd and began meeting with likeminded people who wanted to collaborate and pitch clients as a team. By 2009, MD Becker Partner's boasted a "senior-only" team with collectively more than 25-years of real-world, in-house biotech experience.

The team consisted of me as president and CEO, Janet Dally, senior vice president, and Jeffrey Martini, Ph.D., vice president. Both Jeff and Janet had approached me about joining the firm, as they liked the unique approach. They must have read my initial press release or come across my website, as I had never met either of them before. I couldn't pay any salary or benefits, so we were three independent consultants grouping our time and resources together to set ourselves apart from all the single-shingles. If we signed a client or generated revenue, we divided it among the three of us.

Jeff joined MD Becker Partners with a diverse background in large pharmaceuticals, biotechnology, academic research, and venture capital. Before joining MD Becker Partners, he worked in the Life Science Investment Group at Ben Franklin Technology Partners, which provided direct funding, business assistance and networking opportunities to early-stage and established technology firms throughout Pennsylvania.

Before joining MD Becker Partners, Janet was president of MontRidge, LLC, a boutique investor relations and strategic consulting firm specializing in the life science industry. She first joined MontRidge as vice president in 1998. Before MontRidge, she was vice president of investor relations at Burns McClellan, another life sciences communication firm.

We didn't have an office at first, so we conducted frequent staff meetings at Starbucks in Newtown, Pennsylvania. It was a great location, just off quaint State Street, and offered a beautiful view through all the large windows. However, it was noisy and far from private, with many other groups doing the same thing. One of us would order coffee while the others raced to secure three seats. Jeff, being younger and computer savvy, always brought his MacBook Air laptop to take notes and pull up online research. We'd stay for a few hours depending on the length of our discussion and then return to our homes to continue working separately.

Following in the footsteps of my successful *Beck on Biotech* newsletter, I suggested early on that we create a periodic, online publication and website called the *Life Science Digest* that was launched in January 2009. The articles would be authored by whoever wanted to write or had something relevant to say about a particular biotech topic. Given my penchant for writing, I did the majority of the articles and even brought back my "ASCO-effect" tagline.

The *Life Science Digest* was generating good traffic to our website, which helped increase the firm's visibility. But, of course, it didn't produce any revenue.

"Jeff and Janet," I said one day at Starbucks. "I know things are getting off to a slow start, which means none of us are making any money. But I think if we narrow our focus in specific subsets of the biotechnology sector where others aren't paying much attention, we can stand out better. Knowing that there's a major catalyst on the horizon with the FDA's decision whether or not to approve the first cancer vaccine, Dendreon's Provenge® (sipuleucel-T), one area that I thought fit the description perfectly was cancer vaccines or immunotherapies."

"I think that's a great idea," said Jeff.

"Me too," said Janet.

"Instead of just writing another free article for our *Life Science Digest*, I think we should collaborate on producing a detailed white paper for cancer immunotherapy to help investors, analysts, reporters, and others be better prepared for the great interest in the space soon. We could then charge for the report and help bring in some much-needed cash flow."

"I can contribute to some of the tougher science aspects of the field," said Jeff.

"I can reach out to some key opinion leaders I know, such as Dr. David Berd," replied Janet.

"That's great, and I can also bring in Dr. James Gulley of NIH and Dr. Susan Slovin from MSKCC. Perhaps we could do a virtual 'round-table' discussion with the three of them about the upcoming FDA decision for Provenge and include that as a special section in the document."

Each of us was contributing and working together. We were building something from scratch. It was exciting.

———

I felt that immunotherapies could be poised for dramatic growth as more and more success stories were created, similar to the field of monoclonal antibodies. Monoclonal antibodies were hailed as "magic bullets" when they were developed in the 1970s, only to produce mostly disappointing results for the first ten years of development. Similar to monoclonal antibodies, the early development of cancer vaccines or immunotherapies had proven to be an enormous challenge. In fact, we identified a dozen such programs through our research that had previously failed in late-stage Phase III trials.

While no cancer vaccines were currently approved, the FDA had assigned a Prescription Drug User Fee Act (PDUFA) date of May 1st, 2010, by which time it would respond to Dendreon Corporation's amended Biologics License Application (BLA) for Provenge. Dendreon was seeking licensure for Provenge for men with metastatic castrate-resistant prostate cancer. Anticipation over this event reignited investor interest in the field of active immunotherapy and shares of Dendreon, which traded below $5 in March 2009, had recently hit all-time highs above $40 and the company reached a market capitalization higher than $5 billion.

In early April 2010, MD Becker Partners published its 150-page industry white paper titled "Cancer Vaccine Therapies: Failures and Future Opportunities." It included an overview of the cancer immunotherapy market, interviews with several key opinion leaders (including Dr. Susan Slovin, Dr. James Gulley, and Dr. David Berd), profiles of nearly 40 cancer vaccine companies, and a discussion of the scientific, clinical, and commercial considerations for the major industry participants. We sold the report online for $2,000 a copy, which helped bring in some needed revenue to be split among the three of us. Frankly, it was quite a triumph for the three of us to produce such a comprehensive overview of the space in such a short period. As an electronic report, we didn't make any significant financial investment—just our sweat labor and time. So, each purchase was nearly 100 percent profit.

Beyond Provenge, there were many additional catalysts in 2010 that we believed could ignite further interest in the field of cancer immunotherapy. Nearly 50 clinical programs involving active cancer immunotherapies were currently underway, including almost a dozen that were in pivotal Phase III development with several BLAs planned in 2010.

For example, Bristol-Myers Squibb Company had announced its potential intent to file for regulatory approval for Yervoy® (ipilimumab) in metastatic melanoma in 2010 and had submitted Phase III data for presentation at the ASCO annual meeting being held June 4-8, 2010. Also, GlaxoSmithKline plc was conducting the largest ever Phase III clinical trial in lung cancer treatment with its investigational MAGE-A3 ASCI immunotherapy, with the possibility for data presentation at ASCO 2010.

On April 29th, 2010, the FDA approved Dendreon's Provenge, a cancer vaccine designed to stimulate the immune systems of men with advanced prostate cancer to attack their malignancies. Unlike a prophylactic vaccine, which is given *before* a person gets sick to boost their immune system to fight off infections, this is an example of "therapeutic vaccine," which was designed to attack cancer cells in a person's body. The product was also tailored to each patient by using some of their cells, which created logistical and manufacturing issues.

The approval of the first cancer vaccine generated great interest in the field and our firm's cancer vaccines report. Members of the media, such as Peter Benesh of Investor's Business Daily and Thomas Gryta of Dow Jones Newswires, contacted me as the spokesperson for the report and quoted me in several articles regarding Dendreon.

Beyond Dendreon's Provenge, various immunotherapies were in late-stage clinical development for prostate cancer, including Bavarian Nordic's promising off-the-shelf vaccine set to begin a pivotal Phase III trial in 2010. In fact, our firm identified nine product candidates that were in clinical trials for the treatment of prostate cancer, representing the largest therapeutic disease area within the immunotherapy market.

Bavarian Nordic reached out to our firm to assist the company with generating interest at the upcoming ASCO meeting. The company had recently held another event in Chicago, Illinois on May 6th, 2010, in connection with the BIO Annual Meeting that only attracted approximately eight attendees—significantly below the company's expectations.

MD Becker Partners sent Bavarian Nordic a proposal to run a successful investor meeting for the company in connection with the ASCO annual meeting. The contract was signed the very next day, and the event was scheduled for Saturday, June 5th, 2010, at the Hotel W Chicago City Center, 172 West Adams Street, Chicago, Illinois.

Jeff got married and needed more employment stability than a startup could offer. He ended up leaving MD Becker Partners on May 24th, 2010 to join Cephalon as a medical liaison. I was sad to see him go, especially since I felt like our firm was about to break out, and he had invested a good deal of time. But I understood and respected his rationale and wished him well.

Finding a replacement for Jeff given his unique background and experience at a young age was challenging. Especially since we weren't offering any salary or benefits; just the potential to collaborate on something that might become big someday. As such, we didn't do any active recruiting for his replacement.

Following Jeff's departure, I was nervous that Janet might also decide to leave the firm. Of course, this wasn't the right reason to bring on a partner, but over the summer of 2010 we discussed restructuring MD Becker Partners and making Janet a true partner in the firm, which was formalized in August 2010. Concerning profit-sharing and equity, I had a majority position.

Following a very successful ASCO event, Janet and I had a follow-up teleconference with Bavarian Nordic for ongoing investor relations and public relations work. A formal proposal followed, which the company accepted in September 2010. Bavarian Nordic represented our first major client, and it appeared that the strategy of focusing on cancer immunotherapy was paying off.

In contrast to Dendreon, which was developing a patient-specific prostate cancer vaccine, Bavarian Nordic was developing an "off-the-shelf" prostate cancer vaccine it had acquired when the technology reverted to the NIH following the demise of Therion Biologics.

Dr. James Gulley of the NIH was collaborating with Bavarian Nordic, and we had frequent interactions. We created subsequent events and publications covering the cancer immunotherapy landscape, and it was nice to be working with Dr. Gulley again.

While the future for MD Becker Partners was looking brighter, Lorie went back to work in the autumn of 2010. She taught kindergarten part-time with the hopes of landing a full-time teaching position that would provide better and less costly health insurance coverage than we were able to obtain ourselves. She even worked part-time at Trader Joe's for a while to earn extra money. Whenever our family needed a temporary boost until one of my business ideas succeeded, Lorie was there. I never needed to ask, and she never complained.

"Sometimes even you amaze me," Lorie said during dinner one evening.

"How so?" I asked puzzled.

"While many businesses are struggling to recover from one of the worst recessions, here you are making a success out of a firm you envisioned from day one."

"You know one of my favorite quotes 'behind every good man, there is a great woman,' and it wouldn't have been possible without you."

"It's nice having you working mostly from home. Even the kids have mentioned how much they enjoy when you play catch with a baseball in the backyard after they get home from school."

"Yeah, it's been somewhat of a sad reminder of just how much time I missed with them growing up. But, this is a nice balance now, and I think it has brought us all closer."

"It sure has."

Due to the demands of my previous CEO positions, I was primarily a weekend father. Rosie and Meg did various weekend sports when they were young, including soccer. I would attend their games and even helped as an assistant coach for a season.

But baseball was the sport that connected us through the years. Although we moved to the East Coast, our family remained loyal Chicago Cubs baseball fans. We often went to see them play back in Chicago, including a very chilly and wet opening day game.

We also took family trips to see games when the team was playing within driving distance of our Bucks County home. For instance, we went to see the Cubs play the Pittsburgh Pirates, Philadelphia Phillies, Washington Nationals, and New York Yankees on multiple occasions.

When going to see the Cubs, we usually wore team shirts, caps, and other gear—so we got harassed a lot.

Before one game in Pittsburgh, Lorie was able to get the attention of shortstop Ryan Theriot during the team's warm-up session. After tossing him a ball to sign, he frantically motioned for her to place the cap back on the marker *before* throwing it to him. Ryan was Rosie's favorite player at the time, so she was thrilled to have a signed ball from him!

Another memorable game was when Dad and Linda purchased great tickets for our immediate family to see the Cubs play the Los Angeles Dodgers at Wrigley Field one spring day. We had three generations of Becker present at the early afternoon game, a statement that was briefly displayed on the hand-operated scoreboard through an ad that I had purchased in advance to surprise the family.

Naturally, I was excited when the girls both took an interest in playing baseball. After Rosie and Meg came home from school, I would often take a break from working in my office upstairs. We would go in the backyard to practice batting or play catch.

Meg ended up becoming a darn good catcher in little league. I started calling her Soto after Cubs catcher Geovany Soto, who became the first rookie catcher ever to start on the National League All-Star team. We even got her a Cubs jersey with his name on the back.

Rosie developed quite a good throwing arm from our time playing catch. She could launch a ball from her hand with tremendous speed and accuracy. Often, we would play a game to see how many times we could throw the ball to each other without letting it hit the ground.

"C'mon, put a little pepper on it," I shouted across the yard as she was about to throw the ball to me.

THWOK! One of the sweetest noises in all of the sports; when a baseball hits a leather mitt just perfectly to make that unique sound.

"Nice throw," I said before hurling the ball back to her.

The ball skimmed the top of her glove and bounced over the fence, landing in the Yackel's yard.

"Whoops, what happened there? That throw was perfect," I said. She would amusingly reply with any number of excuses for poor performance on the playing field that I had taught her: The sun was in my eyes, the ball took a bad bounce, the umpire made a bad call, etc.

Going to baseball games and those special summer evenings playing ball in the backyard are among my fondest memories with the girls. That was before they became teenagers when communicating became more difficult and they spent more time with their friends.

Following great success with the 150-page white paper, MD Becker Partners hosted an investor conference focused solely on cancer immunotherapy. The inaugural one-day "Cancer Immunotherapy: A Long-Awaited Reality" conference took place in New York City on October 21st, 2010, at the New York Academy of Medicine.

We invited key opinion leaders, investors, and industry executives to engage in discussions, exchange information, and highlight opportunities in the field of cancer immunotherapy. The ambitious agenda included keynote speakers, panelist and plenary sessions, company presentations, and intimate networking opportunities to meet the needs of all attendees.

The event included a great cast of participants, including a morning keynote address, "The future of cancer vaccine development" by Jill O'Donnell-Tormey, Ph.D., executive director of the Cancer Research Institute. Among the many speakers throughout the day were Dr. James Gulley of NIH and Dr. Susan Slovin of MSKCC. We also had a special introduction by biotechnology legend Stelios Papadopoulos, Ph.D., for the luncheon keynote address, "The challenges for cancer vaccine development in academia and industry" by Martin A. "Mac" Cheever, M.D., principal investigator, Cancer Immunotherapy Trials Network, member & director of solid tumor research at the Fred Hutchinson Cancer Research

Center, and professor of medicine/oncology at the University of Washington.

My opening remarks were brief but served as an important reminder that there is still much work to be done when it comes to treating cancer. I fought back my emotions as I spoke.

"Thank you for coming. It is exciting to have this event at the New York Academy of Medicine location. All of the presenting companies, speakers, attendees—really just a phenomenal turnout for this event. So, a special 'thank you' to all of you for participating and making this such a success."

"I wanted to start off by painting a personal story about cancer as it relates to today's topic. On this date, October 21st, back in 2005, the two middle-aged men shown on the screen embarked on hiking the Appalachian Trail. The objective was that each year we would do a small segment of the trail."

"The first year we did it in 2005, we hiked three different sections along the Delaware Water Gap. We were going to go back in following years to hike other segments of the trail."

"Unfortunately, my dear friend and colleague shown in the prior photo passed away on November 4th of 2006—just over a year later—after being diagnosed with a very aggressive form of sarcoma. So, his path, unfortunately, was changed and so was mine."

"And that gave me a personal interest in the field of cancer therapy. I think there have been a lot of advances, but this is a perfect illustration of how quickly things can change and how the unmet medical need for cancer therapy is a very urgent one."

"I hope from this meeting, one of my personal goals, is that this creates interaction among physicians, investors, key opinion leaders, and everybody with a vested interest in the field of cancer immunotherapy to eradicate this disease."

Sadly, cancer would claim another industry connection less than two months later. On December 16th, 2010, Frank Baldino, Jr. died at the age of 57 from complications related to leukemia, according to a company statement. In August, he had taken a leave of absence from his posts as Cephalon's chairman and chief executive.

At the Franklin Institute in Philadelphia, Pennsylvania, hundreds gathered to pay tribute to Baldino and celebrate his life and accomplishments. Frank was a giant. His force of personality, his vision, the insights he brought to bear made him a rare and gifted leader. The event was packed with scientists, colleagues, friends, admirers, community leaders, and people whose lives he touched.

As I digested the news of Frank's passing, I couldn't help but imagine how my life would have been different if I took his job offer instead of the one from Cytogen. This imaginary speculation was further underscored when Teva

Pharmaceutical Industries Ltd. and Cephalon, Inc. announced in May 2011 that their boards of directors had unanimously approved a definitive agreement under which Teva would acquire all of the outstanding shares of Cephalon for $81 ½ per share in cash, or a total enterprise value of approximately $6.8 billion.

I recalled that shares of Cephalon's stock closed around $45 the day Frank and I had lunch together at the Peacock Inn in Princeton, New Jersey. And now, almost exactly a decade later, Cephalon was being sold for nearly $7 billion while Cytogen had recently disappeared for just over $20 million. Of course, in hindsight, things are apparent that were not from the outset.

Between John Tedesco and Frank Baldino, I was a helpless, frustrated spectator watching cancer cut their lives short. Sure, our family gave to various charities and organizations that supported cancer research. Our kids even setup a lemonade stand to help a childhood friend diagnosed with cancer. But I wanted to do more, yet didn't know how at the time.

———

With our cancer vaccine report, very successful annual immunotherapy conference franchise, and a growing roster of clients, business was finally going well for MD Becker Partners in 2011. By now, we had anywhere from 6-12 active clients at a time and we were working hard to get more. Since the launch of our *Life Science Digest* online portal, we'd published dozens of original articles covering scientific, clinical, and financial aspects of the sector.

In the spring, the FDA approved Yervoy by Bristol-Myers Squibb (BMS) for the treatment of patients with late-stage melanoma. BMS had gained rights to Yervoy through the July 2009 acquisition of Medarex for $16.00 per share in cash, or an aggregate purchase price of $2.4 billion.

Approval of Yervoy was the second victory for the field of cancer immunotherapy within a year. The fact that two different cancer immunotherapies demonstrated improved survival in randomized Phase 3 trials and subsequently were approved by the FDA reignited enthusiasm for the field.

Unfortunately, the celebration didn't last long. Dendreon lost two-thirds of its market value on August 4th, 2011 after abandoning its financial forecast for Provenge. In addition to pulling its projections, Dendreon reported disappointing second-quarter sales and said it would trim expenses and jobs. By Thursday morning, the stock was the subject of a wave of brokerage downgrades.

Dendreon's stock closed down more than 67 percent at $11.69, slashing the value of stakes for investors like S.A.C. Capital Advisors, Vanguard Group, BlackRock Financial Management, and Soros Fund Management, who were among its top 10 shareholders. The decline also hit other biotech stocks, with the major biotech indices off more than 10 percent.

In one of his many early stories covering the cancer immunotherapy field, reporter Bill Berkrot of Reuters quoted me.

"The very fact that Dendreon was unsuccessful in securing a corporate partner either prior to FDA approval or shortly thereafter really underscores the fundamental flaw in their business model," I said, citing the patient-specific nature of the drug, its high price, competition from easier-to-use medicines and Provenge's minimal efficacy.

Dendreon also faced competition from new advanced prostate cancer drug Zytiga® (abiraterone acetate) backed by Johnson & Johnson's marketing muscle, as well as other easier-to-use medicines on the horizon.

Fortunately, Dendreon's woes didn't negatively impact MD Becker Partners. If anything, they helped. Given the fact that we were representing Bavarian Nordic, which theoretically had a better mousetrap when compared to Dendreon's product, we were able to convert many of Dendreon's followers to Bavarian Nordic.

Bavarian Nordic had a compelling story, but I also used my knowledge of Chicago to arrange a popular annual investor gathering for them on top of the city's prestigious John Hancock building each year in connection with the ASCO annual meeting. The events were held at the Signature Room at the 95th®, which boasts what must be the city's best view, with two-story windows all around.

In June 2012, we had an excellent turnout for Bavarian Nordic's event, and it was on this occasion that I first met Brad Loncar, a full-time investor living in Lenexa, Kansas, a suburb of Kansas City. Brad had arrived at the event to learn more about the cancer immunotherapy space since he had a significant position in Dendreon at one point. He managed a family fund that typically consisted of about 40 stocks, nearly half of which were biotech/healthcare. Brad and I were similar in that he was an old-school, buy-and-hold investor who believed the best way to outperform the market is by investing in innovative companies that have great management teams over the long-term. Brad was also a big believer in strong corporate governance and that some companies could be vastly improved by activist investing. He had a lot of admiration for Carl Icahn.

Case in point, Brad sent a widely-publicized open letter to the chairman of Dendreon's board of directors back in February 2011 pleading that the board name one or two outside directors who come from the ranks of shareholders or are outside the ranks of the biotech industry, saying management "are too narrowly focused" and "do not always have shareholder interest in mind."[11] A big part of his complaint was that Dendreon's executives were too bullish about the demand for Provenge and about how fast sales would ramp up.

Not coincidentally, on February 1st, 2012, Dendreon announced that its board of directors had elected John H. Johnson to the position of president and chief executive officer, to succeed Dr. Mitchell H. Gold, who served as president and CEO for nearly a decade. Dr. Gold was elected executive chairman and would serve in that role until June 30th, 2012, at which point he would continue to serve as a director, and Mr. Johnson would become chairman.

Brad got his wish and his stature within the biotech investment community, especially through social media outlets, increased as a result.

———————

Long-term relationships and business partnerships have the potential to be either fantastic or terrible experiences. When relationships are strong, businesses have a much better chance of surviving the challenging times. When business relationships falter, it can result in utter collapse.

Running a company is also stressful. Disagreements are normal and conflicts are not always a problem. But, when thoughts and feelings are not addressed from the start, they can become issues, resentments, crisis, and condemnations.

The specific details of what happened during this period aren't disclosable. But to serve clients more efficiently and effectively going forward, MD Becker Partners was dissolved in May 2013 and Janet and I each formed separate entities that leveraged our respective strengths and backgrounds.

My "new" firm, MDB Communications LLC, got off to a strong start. We divided clients from the former MD Becker Partners, and I also began to sign new customers.

Starting in July of 2014, I came across New York-based biotechnology company Relmada Therapeutics, which was working to addresses unmet needs in central nervous system (CNS) diseases—mostly to treat depression and chronic pain. We had covered the pain therapy sector during some of the past *Life Science Digest* articles, and I also knew about cancer-related pain from my time at Cytogen with its Quadramet product. Relmada was looking to hire a vice president of investor relations and public relations, but I hoped to convince them that outsourcing the function to a firm like MDB Communications would make more sense.

I met with Sergio Traversa, the company's CEO, in New York and we developed excellent rapport. The meetings and phone calls continued throughout the summer, but by October 2014 with no concrete offer or plan, I figured that Relmada wasn't serious about moving forward and dismissed the opportunity.

Instead, on October 6th, 2014, Debbie Hart of BioNJ introduced me to Princeton, New Jersey-based Advaxis, Inc., which was looking for assistance in the areas of investor relations and public relations. After a brief phone conversation, I set up a meeting at Advaxis for Thursday afternoon that same week.

Advaxis was located in the same Forrestal area as Cytogen, so the drive to their office brought back memories of brighter days as CEO.

Attending the meeting was Daniel O'Connor, CEO of Advaxis, Sara Bonstein, the company's CFO, and COO Greg Mayes. We had an enjoyable discussion, and it was clear that we were a good fit for each other. I sent them my standard agreement, which was signed that same day.

Advaxis was particularly well-suited as a client of MDB Communications due to the company's cancer immunotherapy focus. The company's lead Lm Technology™ immunotherapy, axalimogene filolisbac, or AXAL, targets HPV-associated cancers and was in clinical trials for three potential indications: invasive cervical cancer, head and neck cancer, and anal cancer. The company's market capitalization at the time was a mere $50 million.

I hadn't heard anything from Relmada until October 18th, 2014, when I received an offer letter from Sergio for the position of senior vice president, finance and corporate development.

"Honey, you're not going to believe this," I said to Lorie during dinner that evening.

"What's up? Everything okay with your new client?"

"Well, yes and no. I just got an offer letter via email from Sergio at Relmada."

"Seriously? After all this time?"

"I know, can you believe it? Running my consulting business is great, but it would be nice to have colleagues and an office to go to each day, plus a steady salary."

"You know I'm partial towards a steady paycheck. Building and maintaining a consulting client base is such a stress for you—and all of us," she said.

"You've successfully done it twice now between MD Becker Partners and MDB Communications, so you know I'm behind you either way. But, isn't this bad timing? I mean you just signed Advaxis as a client," she added.

"I'm excited about the prospects for both companies, but Sergio hinted that he'd like to promote me to CFO soon and it would also be nice to be back in the C-suite again."

"And what about commuting to New York every day...is there any flexibility with you working from home?"

"No, they were clear that the company and position is based in New York. It can't be that bad, though. Yardley, Pennsylvania is a fairly large commuter town, and a lot of people work in New York."

After a great deal more discussion with Lorie, I decided to accept Relmada's job offer. I was already scheduled to be at Advaxis for an onsite analyst meeting the following week and felt strongly about informing the company of my decision to join Relmada and re-join the biotech industry in person. Accordingly, I planned on asking for some one-on-one time with Dan O'Connor upon arrival.

"Good morning, Dan," I said as he greeted me in the lobby.

"Thanks for coming, Michael. Our guests haven't arrived yet, but they should be here soon."

"That's what I was hoping. Do you have a minute where we could speak privately?"

"Sure, come on back."

Dan escorted me to a nearby empty office and sat off to the side of an unused desk.

"First, I want you to know that I didn't foresee this happening at all, but I interviewed with a biotech company over the summer and after a while just figured that they weren't serious. Much to my surprise, however, they extended me a job offer within days of your hiring me as a consultant for Advaxis.

"It wasn't an easy decision, but I decided to accept their offer. I realize this is terrible form and timing. If there's anything I can do regarding referrals or being available to answer any questions that come up, please know that I want to do whatever it takes to make this right."

I could sense Dan was upset even though he didn't show it. Instead, he was a consummate gentleman.

"Don't worry about it, Michael," he said. "I understand why you decided to take the job and sure; we'll pepper you with questions as they come up. Most of all, I hope it works out for you on every level."

Chapter Eight
Starting Treatment

After many stressful times and associations with New York over the years, I never imagined actually commuting to, or working there. But, much to my surprise, it didn't take me long to embrace the city fully.

The hour-long train ride each way provided some welcome downtime to relax, listen to music, or catch-up on emails. Exploring new restaurants and museums during the lunch hour was also a benefit.

During my first year working at Relmada, I mostly traveled throughout the country to present at various investor conferences and meet with retail investors and brokers. Usually, I went with investor relations director Christine Berni-Silverstein, and we had a lot of fun.

Aside from advancing the company's pipeline of product candidates through clinical trials, employees and investors were focused on Relmada's stock moving to a national exchange from the over-the-counter (OTC) markets. Such a move would help attract a broader, more diverse shareholder base.

The second year working at Relmada was a bit more stressful. In August 2015, the company implemented reverse stock split in an attempt to maintain a minimum closing price of $4.00, one of the requirements for an uplisting to Nasdaq. While not always the case, investors often view a reverse split negatively and opt to sell their shares, sending the share price back down.

Around the same time, Relmada experienced difficulties with Laidlaw & Company Ltd., a United Kingdom-based investment bank that had worked with Relmada since 2011, raising capital and taking the company public via a reverse merger. As part of the payment for its services, Relmada gave Laidlaw a significant stake in the company. Laidlaw, including its two principals, Matthew Eitner and James Ahern, owned about 10 percent of Relmada's common stock. They also suggested two people who were appointed to Relmada's board of directors.

The relationship soured over the years, culminating in a lawsuit by Relmada against Laidlaw in December 2015. Investors hate uncertainty, and with this lawsuit, Relmada was nearly toxic to prospective investors and other investment banks. Relmada's share price fell 43 percent initially, then further yet. The stock price decline adversely affected Relmada's application for listing on the Nasdaq stock exchange, which, in turn, hampered Relmada's ability to raise capital. It made life for Christine and me more difficult.

My personal life was quickly changing with the first day of chemoradiation on January 18th, 2016. As expected, it was bittersweet. On the one hand, nearly two months had passed since finding the suspicious lump on my neck, so it felt great to get started with attacking the cancer finally. The flip side was knowing what lurked around the corner regarding side effects.

The first two days of treatment involved both chemotherapy and radiation, so Lorie and I stayed at the DoubleTree Metropolitan NYC Hotel on Lexington Avenue. We had a quick bite to eat for breakfast at a diner around the corner from the hotel before walking a few blocks to Dr. Pfister's office. The day at MSKCC started at 8:45 am with bloodwork and consultation with nurse practitioner Nicole Leonhart.

"OK," Nicole asked us after reviewing the day's agenda, "any questions?"

I looked at Lorie.

"Not I," she said.

"Me neither," I followed.

"All right then," she said. "What about your plans for getting to and from treatments—will you be staying in the city?"

"Since I work in the city anyway, I'm planning on continuing to commute via train from Pennsylvania."

Nicole's facial expression revealed that this wasn't a viable strategy.

"Do you think commuting will be too difficult?" Lorie asked Nicole.

"Every patient is different, but I wouldn't count on feeling well enough to commute after a few weeks of treatment," Nicole replied. "You should look into some temporary housing here in NYC."

"OK, something to consider," I said.

We returned to the waiting area until a chemotherapy suite became available. Then the fun began with two hours of intravenous fluids, an hour of intravenous anti-nausea medications and kidney protection medication, an hour of intravenous chemotherapy (cisplatin), and then two more hours of intravenous fluids. Of the six-hour total infusion time, four hours were taken up by intravenous fluids flushing out the kidneys, which are at risk for damage from the chemotherapy.

The time passed quickly. Lorie and I chatted throughout, had a small lunch, checked emails, etc. Not quite a day at the spa, but no unpleasant surprises.

The day wasn't over yet. Next was a brief shuttle bus ride to the radiation center for the following component of the therapy. I was told the radiation treatment itself was only about ten minutes, but there was setup time that took up about another hour.

I changed into a cloth gown and stored my items in a locker. Afterward, I sat in a hallway outside of the entrance to the nuclear medicine department waiting to be called back.

"Mr. Becker?" said a nuclear medicine technologist while standing in the doorway.

"Yes, that's me," I replied.

"Great, please follow me."

We walked through a corridor and arrived at my treatment room. Outside of the entrance was a large control center with computer screens showing my treatment plan and images of my head and neck.

Entering the room, I first noticed the giant piece of equipment called a linear accelerator. It is the machine that emits a high energy X-ray beam. My eyes quickly darted to the dreaded radiation mask, which was sitting on a nearby counter. In patients with head-neck cancer treated with IMRT, immobility of the upper part of the body during radiation is usually maintained by a head-neck-shoulder thermoplastic mask.

After lowering the treatment table, a technician instructed me to lay on my back with my head closest to the linear accelerator. He then grabbed my mask from the counter and came back over to me.

"Any particular style of music you would like to hear during treatment?" asked the technician. "Pop, R&B, classic rock..."

"Classic rock," I replied as soon as I heard the option.

"Excellent choice."

Lying supine, the technician began to position my radiation mask, which he then bolted to the treatment table. It fit so tightly that my head and shoulders were completely immobile. Any chance to escape was gone.

"You'll be done in about ten minutes, so just try and relax," said the technician as he exited the room.

Music started playing in the background shortly after he closed the door. Next, I could see and hear the arms of the linear accelerator begin rotating around my trapped body. Despite taking anti-anxiety medication, I was frightened and alone.

A short while later, the machine powered down. The low humming sound it made subsided.

"You're all done, I'll be in momentarily to get you up," said a voice over the intercom.

I didn't feel anything at all during the radiation treatment. The side effects come later, so I left day one feeling emotionally drained but physically fine. The worst part of radiation treatment was that darn mask! The confining nature of the mask and being pinned to the table was more of a mental challenge than anything else.

Tuesday, I woke up early at 5 am feeling wide awake, which could have been a side effect of the steroids they gave me. However, a short while later I started to get a bit nauseous. It was disturbing to see that chemotherapy side effect so soon after treatment, but I took the pill for nausea they prescribed and felt better in about 30 minutes.

Lorie and I stopped for breakfast, and I was able to order my favorite banana toast meal from Bluestone Lane on Lexington in New York and had some coffee as well. We then headed over to MSKCC for day two of chemoradiation.

For the next few weeks, I didn't have to do the 5-6 hour, two-day chemotherapy routine. During that period, I only had daily radiation Monday-Friday. Then, around week three, I went through the same two-day chemotherapy cycle again and the process repeated. The total treatment would last 6-7 weeks.

I continued working at Relmada's office during the majority of the period—spending the usual three hours a day commuting via train between home and NYC on New Jersey Transit. It was grueling, as I was fighting fatigue and nausea and watching nearly everyone around me sneezing and coughing, spreading germs throughout the train cabin.

Lorie and I realized that Nicole was correct; commuting daily for treatment and work was likely going to be too much.

Dad and Linda graciously offered to pay for a temporary apartment in NYC for a few months, which we kindly accepted. Not a cheap solution, essentially like taking on a second mortgage payment, which we couldn't afford to do on our own. But a necessary one—especially when side effects were expected to get progressively worse around week three or four.

After researching various options, Lorie found a suitable one-bedroom apartment through Furnished Quarters. The location was walking distance to both my oncologist and radiation oncologist at MSKCC, which was convenient. We signed a month-to-month agreement.

Moving into an apartment in New York would make a huge difference concerning commuting to work and daily radiation therapy appointments. The most significant downside was not being able to see Lorie and the kids on a regular basis. However, I focused on the relatively short duration of treatment and looked forward to being back home in a few months.

Truth be told, during the entire first week of chemoradiation I felt worse than I had initially expected. I was told the tougher part of therapy would begin around week three or four, so it was disheartening that I felt so awful after only the first round of treatment.

Moments after my brief victory lap for completing the first week of treatment, I started running a fever and felt rundown. A quick call to my oncologist and I was instructed to head over to MSKCC's urgent care facility that night. Fortunately, it was Friday, and both Lorie and Rosie were already in NYC to spend the weekend with me at the apartment. Megan was sick, so she stayed back in Pennsylvania with a friend.

Meteorologists warned of a blizzard that could be the most significant snowstorm in the history of New York City's five boroughs since recordkeeping began in 1869. The snowstorm hadn't hit yet, but the hospital lobby was already reasonably crowded upon our arrival. When I was seen, the nurse took a nasal swab to test for the flu. Everything was fine until the blood test. Sitting in a chair during the blood draw, I felt lightheaded and nauseous, a rare and devastating event for me. As Lorie grabbed me a bucket, suddenly the room went dark.

When my eyes opened, and objects came back into focus, I saw several medical professionals huddled around me. I wanted to ask them what happened, but couldn't since they were busy suctioning vomit from my mouth. Later on, they informed me that I had a vasovagal response, which caused me to pass out and throw up.

Sadly, Rosie was in the waiting area and watched the entire scene unfold. Glancing up from her phone, she noticed a team of nurses rushing to the exam room where I last entered. Next thing Rosie knew, a man lying on a wheeled stretcher was being whisked away. It wasn't until she caught a glimpse of his face that she realized it was me.

Long story short, and despite getting the flu shot that season, the nasal swab came back positive for the flu. The flu effects can be magnified in patients undergoing chemoradiation, which is why I felt so crappy the first week.

Upon diagnosis of the flu, I was immediately placed in an orange hazardous materials-looking outfit with a face mask and put in isolation so as not to get other fragile cancer patients sick. They started me on an antiviral agent Tamiflu® (oseltamivir phosphate), but I needed to stay in the hospital for the full weekend to get IV fluids and rest. Fortunately, I was expected to move forward with starting week two of radiation therapy on Monday with no interruption.

Never a dull moment!

Rattled by the chain of events, Lorie spent Friday night sleeping in a reclining chair next to me at the hospital. I had a private room, but guests still needed to wear disposable gloves, gown, and face mask to minimize spreading the flu. Rosie slept on a couch in a recreation room. Neither location was conducive to a good night's sleep.

Saturday evening, after a substantial snowfall (more than two feet in Central Park), Lorie and Rosie walked back to the apartment to spend the night and get some needed rest.

On the way, they took some time to walk the quiet streets and admire the beauty of the city covered in a blanket of white.

————

In contrast to the first week, the second week of treatment was relatively uneventful. I had daily radiation therapy Monday-Friday, and the effects of the flu seemed to dissipate with each passing day. Still not what I would consider back to 100 percent, but a heck of a lot better than how I felt the prior week!

By now, I'd started to see the same familiar faces in the men's locker room before getting daily radiation at MSKCC. The first few times, there wasn't a lot of discussion or interaction. Slowly, you strike up a conversation that is oddly reminiscent of a prison scene from the movies.

"What are you in for?"

"Where are you from?"

"How long is your sentence?"

Stuff like that. The only thing missing was a harmonica playing sad music in the background.

It was a strange cast of characters. Almost everyone was much older than me. Most of them also had some cancer involvement in the lungs that required surgical removal of at least a portion of them in addition to subsequent radiation.

Then there were the real strange diseases, like the older guy who had cancer in some tissue left behind from his umbilical cord when he was an infant that spread to both his bladder and lungs. Another fellow had cancer of the eye, with visible impact. They all told me they were at peace with their fate—ready to go if this is their time but not minding a more extended stay on this earth if treatment provided the opportunity. Maybe it was because I was the younger one in the crowd, but at that point, I wasn't at all at peace with the situation.

No. I was ready to fight like hell.

At the end of the week, I took the New Jersey Transit evening train heading home to Bucks County, Pennsylvania for the first time since I started treatment. I usually commuted to NYC daily for work, so it was a very familiar ride. But the prospect of seeing my wife and kids, family pets, and sleeping in my bed made the hour and a half trip seem a lot longer— almost like time was standing still.

I planned to spend the weekend home and then return to my apartment in NYC for week three of treatment. It was a calculated risk coming home and being far from MSKCC, especially given what happened last weekend. However, I was fearful that this would be one of the last times that I'd feel up to commuting back-and-forth and I needed a distraction at the moment.

It felt good to wake up in my bed Saturday morning. Absent from the scene was the honking of horns, sanitation trucks, and other city noises from my apartment. In their place was the soothing whisper of a humidifier to help keep my throat from getting dry.

Before I could roll over to embrace Lorie, our pup Gracie hopped into bed and laid down between us—angling for a belly rub. How I missed having our small petting zoo with me in New York. Hank, our Golden Retriever, was not a morning dog and remained asleep in his dog bed on the floor. Favoring Lorie, our Border Collie-German Shepherd mix Addison rested faithfully on the floor by her side of the bed.

Rosie got out of bed around noon and joined me on the large sectional couch downstairs.

"Good morning, or should I say good afternoon?" I joked as she entered the room.

"Good afternoon, how are you feeling?" she replied with a yawn and outstretched arms, still barely awake.

"I'm not feeling too bad so far."

"Great, do you think you might be up to going out for a bit?"

"Hmm, sounds like you have something specific in mind," I replied with a skeptical tone.

"Well, actually I was wondering if you would take me to get a small tattoo," she said awkwardly. "I'm going to be 18-

years old in a few weeks and can get one then on my own. But I'd like you to be there and since you are home..."

"Let me talk to your mother, and we'll see."

Having a few tattoos myself, I knew it would be difficult to say no. Currently wearing a vanity t-shirt that read "World's Greatest Tattooed Dad" didn't help matters either. After a lengthy discussion with Lorie, we made an afternoon appointment for Rosie at The Inkwell in Southampton, Pennsylvania.

Not quite the diversion I was seeking, but I was quite touched that Rosie had selected a tattoo symbolizing me. I always felt that a tattoo should be meaningful and knew this would be something that she wouldn't later regret. Besides, she accompanied me during one of my tattoo appointments and was familiar with the process.

———

The first week of February 2016 marked the beginning of week three for my chemoradiation treatment. By now, the cumulative effects of daily radiation started to appear. Examples included oral mucositis (inflammation of the mucous membranes in the mouth with symptoms ranging from redness to severe ulcerations) and xerostomia (dry mouth).

When I first licensed the North American marketing rights to Caphosol in October 2006, I had no idea that nearly a decade later I would be a customer. The product is intended to treat some of the common side effects of cancer chemotherapy and radiation—both oral mucositis and xerostomia. While these side effects can occur as a result of various treatments, they are particularly prevalent in head and neck cancer patients undergoing chemoradiation like me. The majority of head and neck cancer patients (83 percent) who are receiving radiation therapy develop oral mucositis, and 29 percent develop severe oral mucositis.[12]

It was disheartening that so many years after its commercial introduction, no physician I spoke with had even heard of Caphosol. After a fair amount of nagging and discussion, I was finally able to secure a prescription and locate a nearby pharmacy that carried the product in advance of starting treatment. One the key clinical studies supporting Caphosol's efficacy encouraged using it at the start of therapy. In other words, Caphosol was used before the incidence of oral mucositis or xerostomia as a preventative therapy. The trial demonstrated that Caphosol was able to reduce the severity of oral mucositis, decrease pain and associated use of opioid analgesics, and reduce the days of neutropenia (abnormally low concentration of white blood cells in the blood).[13]

The World Health Organization (WHO) Oral Toxicity Scale measures anatomical, symptomatic, and functional components of oral mucositis. The scale ranges from Grade 0 (no oral mucositis) to Grade 4 (unable to eat solid food or liquids). My current assessment was WHO Grade 2, which meant that I could still eat solid foods despite the presence of ulcers (I only developed one). Caphosol was working, as I never developed additional ulcers or more severe oral mucositis.

I received a progress report during my appointment with Dr. Nancy Lee, my radiation oncologist at MSKCC. The results were encouraging, as the neck lymph node had markedly decreased in size over the first two weeks of therapy—characteristic for my type of cancer. The better news was that the PET imaging study looking at levels of oxygen deficiency (hypoxia) in the tumor tissue showed dramatic improvement. In particular, the pre-treatment scan showed "mild" radiotracer uptake in the primary tumor (right tonsil) and "intense" radiotracer uptake in the neck lymph node, indicating a significant amount of hypoxic tumor cells that are generally more resistant to radiation and many anticancer drugs. However, the most recent PET scan showed "no" radiotracer uptake in the primary tumor and only "mild" persistent uptake in the neck lymph node. Unfortunately, the fact that there was still some hypoxia meant that they wouldn't be able to reduce the amount of radiation to the neck node, which could have minimized some of the side effects.

I had my follow-up hearing test, which showed no change from pre-treatment. Good news, as the chemotherapy can sometimes cause hearing loss.

The start of week four of my chemoradiation treatment involved two days of chemotherapy in addition to my daily radiation treatment. Since I came home for the weekend, Lorie and I took an early morning train into NYC for my chemotherapy appointment on February 8th, 2016. I was feeling some pain that morning from the mouth sore and for the first time in my throat as well. I was miserable the entire train ride but made it to New York, and we headed to MSKCC for treatment.

The day started with radiation therapy, an appointment for blood work, and then a meeting with nurse practitioner Nicole before beginning chemotherapy. Last week when I met with her, she prescribed Neurontin® (gabapentin) and a viscous lidocaine solution to help manage the oral pain. When I communicated my current pain level to her, she also prescribed oxycodone—an opioid medication. After about 30-minutes, the pain was improving and continued to do so throughout the next few hours. Nicole also mentioned that the steroids administered as part of the chemotherapy could help with inflammation and might help alleviate the mouth and throat pain.

My chemotherapy was scheduled for 1 pm, but a routine blood test came back with some unusual readings in the metabolic panel. In fact, had the results been correct, the nurse said my heart would likely have stopped! They couldn't proceed with chemotherapy if the results were accurate. So, they needed to take another blood test to determine whether or not the readings were correct. Not surprisingly, the first results were wrong and the second set was perfectly normal. As a result, the chemotherapy treatment proceeded, but not until around 2:30 pm.

I finally finished chemotherapy at 7:45 pm. Lorie and I went to Jackson Hole, a nearby restaurant for a late dinner before heading back to the apartment. The second dose of oxycodone left me feeling little pain, and I had an appetite. It was the first time I felt comfortable going out to eat in more than three weeks. For some odd reason, the French toast was the only thing that sounded good on the menu and had some much-needed calories. I ate the entire portion except for some of the crust. It was a fantastic end to a day that started off a little rough.

After the second day of chemotherapy, Lorie returned home on Tuesday, and I stayed in the apartment to continue daily radiation and work. I was nervous how I would handle this second cycle of chemotherapy as opposed to the first round when I came down with the flu.

The week was uneventful, with increased taste alteration and fatigue being the most prominent changes I noticed. My heart rate and blood pressure were elevated, so my physician ordered an extra 2-hour intravenous hydration session. Frankly, I was happy to do so, as I planned on coming home to Pennsylvania for another extended weekend.

Sunday was Lorie's 50th birthday in addition to being Valentine's Day, which is why I wanted to make it home. I owed her a proper celebration after we got past my cancer treatment, but in the meantime, it would be nice to have a small party at home.

Before taking the train home on Friday afternoon, I managed to make it over to Bloomingdale's in New York and got her a Pandora necklace that I knew she'd like along with a card.

I took the train home on Friday afternoon but spent most of the day on Saturday sleeping. It wasn't like me at all. I'm generally not one to take naps, but the fatigue from radiation and chemotherapy made it hard even to keep my eyes open at times. I felt like I was sleeping the entire weekend away!

On Sunday, Lorie was shocked that I managed to find time to shop for her in my condition, but her milestone birthday was too essential to pass up. She enjoyed the necklace almost as much as our favorite ice cream cake from Halo Pub in Princeton, New Jersey. According to Lorie, no birthday is complete without cake.

From what the doctors told me, week five of chemoradiation would be when things start to get a little rough with the treatment. Accordingly, I was a bit nervous about what the coming days and weeks would bring.

Knowing that my condition would likely start to deteriorate, February 12th, 2016 marked Lorie's last day at school for six weeks under the Family and Medical Leave Act of 1993 (FMLA), a United States federal law requiring covered employers to provide employees with job-protected and unpaid leave for qualified medical and family reasons. It allowed her to spend more time with me at the apartment in NYC.

Sure enough, another common side effect of chemoradiation treatment emerged during week five—a skin condition called radiation dermatitis. Just like oral mucositis, radiation dermatitis is graded on a scale, with Grade 1 being mild and Grade 4 being severe. In most patients, radiation dermatitis is mild to moderate (grades 1 and 2), but 20–25 percent of patients experience severe reactions.

At the time, I had mild to moderate radiation dermatitis on my neck in the area that was being targeted. It is characterized by mild erythema (red rash), which could easily be mistaken for an acute sunburn. The more severe forms of radiation dermatitis are associated with itchy, peeling skin and ultimately open wounds and ulceration. I was hoping that my condition didn't advance to those stages.

The treatment for radiation dermatitis is keeping the skin moist by applying moisture-retentive, barrier products such as Aquaphor® ointment. No creams or lotions have shown superior efficacy over another in randomized clinical trials. This includes topical steroids and other agents.

Other than that, there was some indication that my kidney function might be impaired due to elevated serum creatinine levels. Cisplatin, the chemotherapy I receive, is primarily excreted by the kidneys and has been associated with an increased risk of kidney damage.[14] Creatinine is a waste product from the normal breakdown of muscle tissue. As creatinine is produced, it's typically filtered through the kidneys and excreted in urine. Doctors measure the blood creatinine level as a test of kidney function and dehydration.

I ended up having intravenous hydration with saline and potassium to flush out the kidneys and felt pretty good afterward. Fatigue was still my major complaint, but also par for the course.

My medical team wanted to do additional hydration Friday late afternoon. However, that would have interfered with my getting back to Pennsylvania in time to see Megan that night before her freshman formal dance. While perhaps insignificant in the grand scheme of things, I couldn't help but wonder if this would be one of the last times I would see Megan all dressed up and dating. After explaining the situation, a nurse at MSKCC came up with the solution of hydrating me on Saturday instead.

Our friend and fellow photographer Sharon Mastrosimone was kind enough to come over to our home that evening and take pictures before Megan's dance. Despite the glistening red rash around my neck, Sharon's photographs made the night worthwhile.

Even one of our twin tuxedo cats, Dolce and Gabbana, made it into the pictures with their stark black and white markings resembling men's formal wear.

"We'll name our child Gabbana," Megan jokingly stated to her date as she cradled her favorite feline like a newborn baby in her arms. The resulting photo was worthy of a proper birth announcement.

The next morning, Lorie and I returned to New York instead of spending the weekend back home in Pennsylvania. I spent Saturday afternoon at MSKCC with Lorie getting hydration, but I did it with a smile on my face looking at pictures from the prior night on my phone. Megan looked so beautiful and grown up. I was glad that I got to be there with her.

Week six was relatively uneventful—at least as it related to my cancer treatment. The regular hydration during the week lowered my creatinine levels, which correlated with improving kidney function.

In fact, the most significant issue for me this past week was throwing out my back. It happened on occasion before I had cancer. But since back pain can also be a sign of kidney issues, I was instructed once again to make a trip over to the urgent care center at MSKCC. By this point, I felt like I should be enrolled in some frequent-flyer program to accumulate points for my numerous urgent care visits.

Fortunately, all the diagnostic tests came back fine. They prescribed pain medication and a muscle relaxer. Once the drugs kicked in, I fell sound asleep sitting up on a gurney. I must have been in the middle of reading email messages, as I still had my phone in one hand.

"Always working," Lorie chuckled as she took a quick photo with her phone.

The likely culprit for my back pain was the mattress in our temporary apartment which was a good deal softer than the one we had back at home. The folks at Furnished Quarters were great during our stay, and they promptly replaced the mattress when we asked.

Throughout treatment, I made it to work as often as physically possible. It was a quick subway or cab ride to the office. On rare occasions, such as having back problems, I worked remotely from the apartment via computer and was always in touch with the office through email, text, and phone conversations.

There's a big difference between *wanting* and *needing* to continue working. Maintaining income and health insurance are significant reasons why some cancer patients need to stay on the job. I continued to work mainly because I felt well enough to do so, appreciated the routine of my day, and valued the distraction. Besides, our family's health insurance was through Lorie's employer.

Everyone at Relmada was incredibly supportive, trying to get me to eat by offering food or supplements. Christine would always do her best to keep me hydrated, bringing many coconut and other electrolyte drinks for me to try. I found the support and friendship of my co-workers helpful.

For the first time, I understood why John Tedesco needed to stay so connected to Cytogen during his disease. As a cancer patient, you don't want to feel useless. That only reinforces the negativity of the disease. The more normal, day-to-day activities that you can do help provide a sense of self-worth and a feeling that *you* are still the one in control, not cancer. Going to the office, being on conference calls, all of it provided a sense of normalcy and distraction. Unlike John, however, I was fortunate to have temporary residence close to both work and MSKCC, which made it much easier for me to manage the commute.

———————

At long last, Monday, February 29th, 2016 marked the beginning of my final week of chemoradiation. The previous evening, however, I started running a temperature of 102 degrees Fahrenheit that prompted my second trip to the urgent care center at MSKCC over the weekend. The apparent concerns being influenza, bacterial infection, etc. that could delay my final cycle of chemotherapy.

After a variety of tests, influenza and infection were ruled out. While it is possible to run a low-grade temperature from daily radiation, a high temperature such as mine was unexpected. It left everyone wondering what was causing my fever and why it was so high. Since there was no immediate cause for concern, they decided not to admit me overnight and said that I could use acetaminophen to reduce the fever. But they acknowledged that it was unlikely I'd be receiving chemotherapy the next day.

On Monday, we saw Nicole at MSKCC and could tell that she was on the fence about proceeding with chemotherapy, given that my temperature was again above 100.4 degrees Fahrenheit. She conferred with Dr. Pfister, and they opted to be cautious and postpone treatment for twenty-four hours. The only good news was they did not expect this delay to change my final day of chemoradiation therapy, which was that Friday.

Around the time of my daily radiation treatment in the afternoon, my temperature had dropped to low grade, and I was hopeful that I could continue with chemotherapy the next morning.

My lower back pain continued to be a problem, so I was prescribed a fentanyl transdermal skin patch—a stronger opioid medication. I'm not talking minor pain or discomfort, but debilitating pain that made it difficult to get out of bed or rise from a sitting position. I had experienced lower back pain issues in the past, but they usually only lasted a day or two and weren't nearly this severe.

Sure enough, I was able to continue with my final doses of chemo on Tuesday and Wednesday. On the last day of chemotherapy, I was joined not only by Lorie but also Megan. She was chaperoned on the trip to NYC by Lorie's best friend since 3rd grade of elementary school, Debby Novack, who came into town to help out. Not an overly exciting day for Megan—sitting around the chemotherapy suite and shuffling between various appointments—but it was great having her there.

It was bittersweet watching the final drops of cisplatin fall from the bag, stream down the winding tubes, and finally, enter the intravenous line into my vein.

On the positive side, I was able to complete all of the three cycles of chemotherapy that are associated with the encouraging survival rates published by the physicians at MSKCC. Some patients don't make it through all three cycles due to side effects, and I'd been nervous earlier that week when I started running a fever. Skipping the last cycle had been discussed as a possibility.

On the negative side, the week following chemotherapy was typically tricky for me regarding nausea and a general sense of feeling crappy. On top of that, the medical team reminded me that the coming few weeks would be the toughest. They indicated this was due to the cumulative effects of both radiation and chemotherapy, as the two therapies continue to exert their toxic effects even after they are discontinued.

The following two days (Thursday and Friday) were also my final days of radiation therapy and marked the end of my seven-week chemoradiation therapy journey. I was looking forward to having at least part of my life back next week—not being a slave to the daily treatments and chemotherapy cycles. Any remaining doctor appointments would be routine checkups leading up to a PET scan in approximately 3-4 months to determine in part whether or not the treatment was successful or if further intervention was needed.

My lower back pain subsided, and I could get up and down much better than even a few days ago. Either the muscle spasm went away on its own, or the myriad of pain medicines and muscle relaxers finally started working. Regardless, I was happy and better positioned to deal with the coming weeks with one less ailment to worry about.

On Friday, I was informed that I could take the dreaded radiation mask home with me. I no longer needed to wear the mask for daily radiation therapy, which made me *very* happy.

Lenny, one of the nuclear medicine technicians at MSKCC, told me what some of the other patients did with their masks after their radiation treatment was done.

"Some make decorative items, such as flower pots, out of them. Another patient burned his mask in a sadistic revenge ceremony," he said.

"Hmm, that last option has a certain type of appeal for me," I confessed.

It conjured up thoughts of Darth Vader's helmet, last seen burning in a funeral pyre in the movie *The Return of the Jedi* before winding up in the hands of Kylo Ren in *Star Wars: The Force Awakens*.

Setting aside fantasizing about how to destroy my radiation mask, I enjoyed certain freedom knowing that I was no longer beholden to a daily treatment schedule. I also took comfort that I received the very best treatment possible for my disease by the entire team at MSKCC. It's amazing how quickly the seven-week treatment cycle passed, and it all seemed like a blur now.

While I never looked forward to the daily radiation treatment, it was at least a constant reminder that I was doing something to treat the disease. Now I had that same empty feeling that plagued me when I was first diagnosed and searching for the best treatment—the sense that I *should* be actively doing something but wasn't.

By the second week of March 2016, I was able to move out of my temporary apartment in New York and return home to Bucks County, Pennsylvania. I don't know whether it was being away from the loud traffic noises or just finally sleeping in my bed, but the first night home was the best night's sleep I had in weeks.

As predicted by my medical team, the weeks following chemoradiation were the most difficult due to the delayed toxic effects of therapy. For me, week eight was the worst, and I required additional hydration pretty much every other day during that week. My electrolyte levels, in particular, magnesium, were low. Fatigue was probably the most significant side effect, but in general, I just felt like I had a nasty case of the flu.

My salivary output and taste buds were still off as a lingering effect from the chemoradiation therapy, although I was told they should return over time. It made it difficult to eat, or at least find food that was appealing. I lost more than 20 pounds since the start of treatment, which didn't disappoint me as much as it did my doctors.

A post-treatment visit with Dr. Nancy Lee was scheduled for mid-May 2016, which is when I expected to get my first update on the treatment efficacy. She did order a PET scan on my last day of treatment, which looked encouraging although it's difficult to draw any definitive conclusions at that early stage. Nonetheless, there was decreased fluorodeoxyglucose (FDG) uptake in the right tonsil and the rim corresponding to the neck node. Interestingly, the neck node also initially measured 4.0 x 2.6 centimeters and now measured 2.3 x 1.6 centimeters, which was a dramatic decrease in size.

I returned to work full-time around mid-March 2016, which meant getting up early and commuting via train to New York again. The radiation burn marks on my neck were nearly gone, and you'd hardly know by looking at me that I just went through seven weeks of pure unadulterated hell. Fatigue was still an issue, although it improved slightly with each passing day.

Unfortunately, the litigation between Relmada and Laidlaw was ongoing and still draining the company's financial resources. I was monitoring the cash situation and knew that

Relmada had enough capital to maintain its day-to-day operations for some time.

By the end of May 2016, my weight declined by a total of 30 pounds since the start of chemoradiation. My taste buds were now 80-90 percent back to normal and "most" foods tasted the same as before therapy. Unfortunately, my saliva output was still way down, so eating dry foods like crackers or bread, was very challenging. I managed to eat a hamburger by taking off the top bun and eating the rest with a fork and knife along with a hefty amount of ketchup.

The most significant problem was my general lack of interest in eating, which I initially thought was due to the taste disturbances. Most days I had a high protein, nutritional shake for both breakfast and lunch and then a "normal" dinner and dessert. I hadn't been out to a restaurant since much earlier in therapy since I was self-conscious about my slower eating habits.

Until recently, I would come home and pass out on the couch from exhaustion at the end of the workday. Now, I was able to stay awake through dinner, watch some television, and go to bed at a reasonable hour. I still slept on the morning train ride to New York and looked forward to the weekends where I usually slept until noon or later to catch up on rest.

The one major issue I tried to ignore was the psychological impact of being a cancer survivor—namely depression. Societal expectations have taught men not to display emotions. We're trained from an early age to be confident, stoic, and strong. It was tough to fulfill this role or expectation as a male cancer survivor. On more than one occasion I burst into an emotional crying session lasting a good 15-minutes. I'm not talking about the quiet episode of crying with sniffles and a tear or two down the side of your cheek. I mean full-fledged bawling your eyes out accompanied by nasal discharge and the near inability to speak normally.

"I...I...I...nuh...na," I'd cry out, "need a tissue."

The first such crying breakdown occurred around the start of chemoradiation when my wife and Rosie first came to my temporary apartment in New York. In retrospect, I had bottled up all of the emotion from first discovering the growth on my neck, to receiving a formal cancer diagnosis, to my first infusion of chemotherapy—and let it all out at once.

I don't think I've ever cried as long, loud, or hard in my entire life. I wanted so badly to be strong in front of both Lorie and Rosie. Evidenced by the blank stares on their faces as they tried desperately to comfort me, I know neither of them expected the emotional outburst.

On another occasion, I broke down alone after showering the morning of Rosie's senior prom. I had started to think about how happy I was to get home from New York during therapy to see Megan for her freshman formal and recalled the photographs from that evening with my neck visibly red from the radiation therapy. Then I started to think, are these going to be the last "big" events I will be around to see for each of my daughters? That spiraled into a series of awful "what if" questions that left me again in a giant puddle.

Most of the time I was able to maintain a positive outlook and not let cancer "win" by occupying my every thought, in part thanks to the medications prescribed by Dr. Jeffrey Freedman, my psychiatrist at MSKCC. Staying positive was made harder by the requirement for periodic tests and imaging studies to determine whether or not cancer has returned. Even aside from those regular tests, it felt like I was always watching over my shoulder for signs or symptoms of cancer's return.

In early May, for example, Lorie noticed that my voice had changed. At first, she dismissed it as that froggy, lower tone you sometimes get first thing in the morning or when you have a head cold. But it didn't go away, and eventually, even I noticed it. Subsequently, I found that the neck area under my chin seemed a bit swollen.

Stranger yet, Gracie started spending an unusual amount of time with her snout very close to the right side of my right throat, sniffing intently. It would have been easier to dismiss had Gracie not started doing the same thing leading up to my original diagnosis. Her behavior stopped after I finished initial treatment.

My first thought was "#@$&!" cancer had now spread to the vocal cords, the larynx (or voice box), or other areas of the throat.

During an appointment with my head and neck surgeon, he didn't see anything suspicious upon visual examination. His initial diagnosis was that the voice change and neck swelling were merely some of the after-effects of radiation therapy, which can manifest even months after treatment. Nonetheless, he wanted to confer with both my medical oncologist and radiation oncologist to determine whether or not an imaging study was warranted.

In the meantime, I tried to adjust to my new bass-baritone "Barry White" voice...which I was told may or may not return to normal. The next major event would be my PET scan scheduled for July 19th, 2016, which would be the first such imaging test following treatment.

Much to my surprise, I received a call back from MSKCC after the Memorial Day holiday stating that they wanted to move up the date for my first post-therapy PET scan. It was rescheduled for Friday, June 3rd, 2016, which meant that I wouldn't receive a phone call with the results until the following Monday.

For head and neck cancer, this first PET scan following chemoradiation therapy is a big deal. Based on long-term follow-up in a large uniform cohort at MSKCC, a "complete response" to therapy, defined as no evidence of disease on clinical examination and post-treatment PET, is associated with a five-year overall survival rate of 79.8 percent. In contrast, for patients with a suspected "incomplete response" on the first PET scan, the 5-year overall survival rate dropped to 57.0 percent in the same study.[15]

After a long, anxious weekend my PET scan results were worth the wait. The report couldn't have been better. There was *no* accumulation of the radiotracer in my tonsil, the previously enlarged lymph node, vocal cords, or any other area of concern in my head and neck area. Sometimes inflammation and other artifacts from treatment make it difficult for radiologists to completely rule out residual disease and therefore cautious language can be used in the radiology report, which wasn't the case for me. Additionally, there was a marked decrease in the size of the infected lymph node.

Personally, I'm not a fan of the terms "cure" or "cancer free" since there is no way for doctors to know with certainty that all of the cancer cells in my body are gone. In fact, some cancer cells can remain unnoticed in the body for years after treatment. So, I preferred to embrace the phrase "no evidence of disease," which references the disappearance of all signs of cancer in response to treatment.

If cancer does return, it often happens within the five years following the first diagnosis and treatment. In this regard, I was optimistic about the expected 80 percent 5-year survival rate—especially when compared to some other aggressive cancers, such as pancreatic cancer, which is associated with a 5-year survival rate of only 6 percent.[16]

I tried to digest the positive news and looked forward to slowly regaining some control over my life. Fatigue was largely gone, I was gaining weight, and saliva output was increasing. I even started to resume my weekend pursuits like photography. My work was beginning to be published in a variety of magazine outlets, and I was happy to have renewed this creative outlet.

Back at the office, I was recently promoted to CFO of Relmada and took on the role by drinking from a proverbial fire hose. I first joined Relmada in 2014 as senior vice president of finance and corporate development. In my new position, however, I was responsible for all corporate finance and accounting activities for the company.

Relmada's fiscal year ended June 30th, so there was a sense of urgency to complete a variety of required activities and regulatory filings. Unfortunately, everyone in the finance department left before my promotion, and there was little in terms of transitional materials or instruction.

I had to figure everything out on my own and search through various electronic folders, files, and emails to make sense of it all. It was a daunting task. Even so, with the help of our accounting and bookkeeping firms, we were able to complete Relmada's annual SEC report and filed it on schedule.

It felt nice to be back in the "C-Suite" again, although the distraction of the company's ongoing lawsuit with Laidlaw still made raising capital very difficult and Relmada's cash was running low.

———

In early June 2016, with only one opioid tablet left in my prescription bottle, I felt that fate was telling me it was time to get off the drug. I wasn't experiencing as much pain as before, so it made sense to forgo refilling my prescription and just quit.

I took my last pill on a Thursday and was scheduled to photograph a Bar Mitzvah event for a neighborhood friend that Saturday. I didn't sleep well at all on Friday night, so Saturday wasn't off to a good start. By the time the event was over, I was feeling horrible. I was restless, anxious, and sweating excessively.

After not sleeping at all again on Saturday night, I was edgy and started to experience both nausea and diarrhea. I finally asked Lorie to take me to the emergency room at St. Mary's Hospital.

Although the local hospital had my medical records and knew I was a cancer patient, the topic of opioid withdrawal never came up. And frankly, it didn't occur to me either. They gave me some medication to alleviate the symptoms and sent me home after not finding anything medically wrong.

When we got home, I went straight to my computer and started searching the Internet for my symptoms and was shocked to see that they were all there: a headache, nausea, sweating, anxiety, pervasive fatigue, depression, restlessness. And the one thing that caused such ailments—sudden opioid withdrawal. Quitting cold turkey.

"Lorie," I called out to her sheepishly. "I think I found out what my problem is..."

"Okay, what?"

"All of my symptoms point to opioid withdrawal, and I took my last pill on Thursday, so I'm thinking..."

"Wait. You did what? Did you stop taking that medication without tapering? You're supposed to be the biotech guru who knows all about medicine. Why didn't you say something! Even I know you need to taper off opioids."

"I thought that the withdrawal symptoms would be craving another pill the next day and having to battle that kind of demon. I never thought there were all these other side-effects, especially the anxiety and depression, fatigue, and inability to sleep."

"Sometimes, you still surprise me, Michael," she said with a laugh. "And not always in a good way."

As someone familiar with the opioid market, especially given Relmada's pain-focused product pipeline, the fact that I didn't consider tapering off the medication was inexcusable. I received a four-week tapering schedule that started me back on the last opioid dose level I was on, then gradually declining to zero tablets by the end of June 2016.

I felt that I had gone through hell already and that the worst was undoubtedly over, so going back on the opioid seemed counterintuitive. However, I followed the tapering schedule and was able to sleep for the first night in more than four days. All of the other symptoms went away within a day. I was done with the opioids before the end of the month without further issue.

Nonetheless, my personal experience shows that opioid addiction danger is real. I had only used oxycodone for a few months and didn't consider myself an addict. I knew about the drug's side effects, such as constipation, mental clouding, upper gastrointestinal symptoms and more. I didn't consider addiction as a risk over a matter of months.

By taking opioids for a few months, I had increased my daily dose during this period due to tolerance. The opioid signaling system has a remarkable ability for tolerance development. Although not all patients necessarily develop profound tolerance, in many cases doses have to be increased over time to maintain the same analgesic benefit. The result is an addiction—and it could happen to just about anyone. In fact, tolerance can develop in a matter of hours depending on the opioid dose being used.

Historically, physicians prescribed opioids only at the end of life or terminal disease setting. Such patients never really had enough time to develop tolerance or experience addiction. Nowadays, patients are prescribed opioids to treat chronic pain and other conditions that result in more prolonged use, which increases the risk of becoming addicted.

In late July 2016, as I approached the five-month mark since completing chemoradiation, I could finally start to see the light at the end of the tunnel. Just that month, I began to notice a significant improvement in both energy and ambition.

I went to movies, ran errands, did a photoshoot, and even jump-started our car. It seemed like a miracle! Before that, my weekend activities consisted solely of laying on the couch napping or watching television after managing to get through the exhausting work week routine.

I'm not sure if the increased energy was related to my body finally starting to heal or the fact that a few weeks prior I had started taking a particular type of ginseng supplement that has been shown to help with cancer treatment-related fatigue. Either way, the difference was dramatic compared to a month ago.

Unfortunately, my appetite wasn't quite back to normal, and my weight was now down a total of 46 pounds from the start of therapy. Don't get me wrong, I was thrilled to have shed those unwanted pounds, but I don't think the chemoradiation diet fad will catch on anytime soon. Aside from not being hungry, my saliva output was still diminished, and that impacted on food selection and taste.

However, with the recent favorable PET scan, energy returning, and being back to what I considered my ideal weight, you'd think the word "cancer" would slowly start to fade from everyday thoughts and discussion. Not so.

Case in point: A series of minor gastrointestinal issues were easy to dismiss until I was vomiting for the fifth time one evening. After briefly passing out while making my way to the bathroom, Lorie had to call 911. I couldn't imagine any possible connection between cancer and the new gastrointestinal symptoms. But it didn't stop me from going to that "dark place" while lying face down on the bathroom floor in my own vomit and during my first ambulance ride to the hospital (not as exciting as it seems on television).

Fortunately, this was one of the few non-cancer related trips to the emergency room. I was diagnosed with the norovirus, also known as the winter vomiting bug. Lucky me to catch such a bug during the middle of summer! After receiving two bags of intravenous solution to replenish my electrolytes, I was released with some anti-nausea medication and felt much better by Monday.

What I hear from other cancer survivors is true—every little ache or anything out of the ordinary immediately causes anxiety that the disease has somehow returned. You are always looking over your shoulder.

Fortunately, the rest of the summer was uneventful concerning medical issues. And in October 2016, Lorie and I witnessed a truly incredible sight. Something that many people never imagined seeing in their lifetimes. The Chicago Cubs baseball team won the World Series for the first time in 108 years. As native Chicagoans, we both had so many relatives who would have loved to see this event. I felt so blessed that it happened in my lifetime.

My brother-in-law, Mark, even tried to coerce me into meeting him in Cleveland for game seven of the fantastic series with the Indians. Under any other circumstance, I would have jumped at the opportunity. Unfortunately, I knew that I just wasn't physically up for such an adventure. I was quite content to watch with Lorie from the comfort of our couch, and we saw the entire game. It was truly magical.

Later that month, I was invited by Brad Loncar to ring the Nasdaq Stock Market Opening Bell to celebrate cancer immunotherapy advances and the one-year listing anniversary of his Loncar Cancer Immunotherapy exchange-traded fund. During the spectacular event, I got to see a lot of familiar faces, such as Dan O'Connor from Advaxis, who wished me well in my fight against cancer.

As the Nasdaq opening countdown progressed, I thought back to happier days when Lorie and the kids were with me doing the market opening for Cytogen. I also thought about the following month; time again for my favorite Thanksgiving meal. Sadly, our wonderful neighbors, Sue and Roger Yackel, moved out of state a few months before to be closer to their children. There would be no grand Yackel feast this year.

But I was thankful for so very much during that time. The encouraging PET scan over the summer, the promotion at work to CFO, and my energy and overall health slowly returning. It was all exactly as I had hoped—the chemoradiation treatment was brutal, but becoming a distant memory with the prospect of now being free of cancer.

Chapter Nine
Recurrence

While my next PET scan was scheduled for early February 2017, radiation oncologist Dr. Nancy Lee wanted to keep the intervals consistent at six months. As a result, MSKCC moved the date for my PET scan up to December 14th, 2016. The previous, encouraging PET scan was done in June 2016.

Unfortunately, the latest PET scan contained terrible news. Multiple new spots consistent with malignancy showed up that were not visible six months ago. This included activity in lung nodules, subcarinal/left hilar lymph nodes (near the trachea), and mild activity around the tonsils and in the region of the oral cavity. A subsequent CT scan confirmed the results.

In the world of medicine, however, cancer doesn't exist until the abnormal cells are viewed under a microscope.

Accordingly, I needed to have a biopsy taken from one or more of the suspicious areas highlighted on the PET scan. I didn't need to wait for that procedure and the subsequent results to know the outcome.

For head and neck squamous cell carcinoma, which was my initial diagnosis, lungs represent the most frequent site of cancer spread and account for 66 percent of distant metastases.[17] This information, combined with the imaging results, left very little chance that the biopsy results would be benign.

I also couldn't help but think back to when Gracie was curiously sniffing around my neck area in May. If only she could have verbalized what her canine senses picked up at the time.

Early morning on December 23rd, 2016, I had my biopsy consultation with Dr. Bernard Park, surgeon and deputy chief of clinical affairs, thoracic service at MSKCC in New York. During the meeting, he presented the pros and cons of a couple of scenarios. Lorie and I both felt like we were in excellent hands, since he took care to explain all the details and why he was leaning towards performing a bronchoscopy.

"If I do a bronchoscopy," Dr. Park said, "I can look down your airway through a thin viewing instrument called a bronchoscope. The bronchoscopy requires general anesthesia, so you'll be out during the procedure."

"During the procedure, I can remove tissue from the suspicious lymph node, and if I think we got a decent tissue sample, then we're done with the biopsy portion."

"That's it?" I asked.

"Right," he replied. "But the second option is a wedge resection, during which I'd remove a portion of your lung around one of the suspicious nodules that showed up on the PET scan. It is an inpatient procedure and may include several days in the hospital since there is a chance of puncturing the lung."

"That sounds a lot riskier. Is one option better than the other?" Lorie asked.

"Either would be fine," he said. "But here's what we'll do, I'll begin with the bronchoscopy and *only* do the wedge resection if I'm uncomfortable that we didn't get enough tissue from the bronchoscopy. I don't want to do the bronchoscopy and see that it won't work for our biopsy purposes and then have to schedule you for the second procedure and possibly delay results."

"OK," I said. "That sounds like a great approach. I guess I'll just wake-up after the procedure and see which way things went."

We scheduled the biopsy procedure for Thursday, December 29th, 2016. Lorie and I stayed overnight in NYC on Wednesday since my appointment at MSKCC was scheduled to start at 9:15 am.

Fortunately, Dr. Park was able to get sufficient tissue from the suspicious lymph node via the bronchoscopy procedure, and he didn't need to do the surgical resection to go after the other nodules in my lungs. The formal biopsy results would take a few days, but Dr. Park spoke to us with a sad clarity shortly after the procedure.

"The node tissue didn't look healthy," he said. "And given that disease progression to the lungs is relatively common in advanced head and neck cancer, in my opinion, the biopsy will most likely confirm the spread of original cancer to the lungs. Or, it could just be an unrelated new lung cancer just showing up now—but that would be rare."

If confirmed by the biopsy results, it would mean a cure is no longer an option. My diagnosis would shift to terminal disease—no effective treatment exists. I was devastated, and so was Lorie.

———

2017 wasn't off to a stellar start.

During the follow-up appointment with my oncologist at MSKCC, we received disappointing news that the biopsy of my chest lymph node contained the same cancer cells (squamous cell carcinoma) as the original tumor in my tonsil. Cancer initially confined to my head and neck had spread below my collarbone to distant sites.

Dr. Pfister proceeded to discuss potential treatment options, including a clinical trial at MSKCC involving Bristol-Myers Squibb's Opdivo® (nivolumab), a type of immunotherapy called a checkpoint inhibitor. The body's immune system has a braking mechanism, a "checkpoint" to prevent immune responses against normal body cells. Cancer cells can hijack checkpoint proteins, such as programmed death-1 (PD-1), to avoid being identified and eliminated by the immune system. However, when these checkpoint proteins are blocked, the "brakes" on the immune system are released, and the body is better able to kill cancer cells.

Assuming that I met the study criteria, I was expected to start treatment the following week. While the FDA already approved Opdivo as a treatment for recurrent head and neck cancer, the clinical study would evaluate whether or not adding targeted radiation directed at one single lung tumor could improve outcomes.

I was already familiar with the synergy between radiation and other forms of therapy, especially immunotherapy. Coincidentally, we were exploring such synergies back at Cytogen with the company's Quadramet being combined with the prostate cancer vaccine being developed by Dr. Gulley at the NIH. Small world.

As the MSKCC trial was randomized, however, I might or might not be one of the patients to receive the potential added benefit of the radiation therapy. Such uncertainty troubled me. However, patients in both arms of the trial received Opdivo, so I'd at least get an active drug in recurrent head and neck cancer in either case.

By chance, I was familiar with checkpoint inhibitors and wrote about enthusiasm for the drug class in a July 8th, 2013 article for my firm's *Life Science Digest* publication. In addition, a research report titled "Immunotherapy – The Beginning of the End for Cancer" issued by analysts at U.S. bank Citigroup on May 22nd, 2013, boldly predicted that the annual market for immunotherapies—defined as including checkpoint agents, vaccines and cell therapy—would exceed $35 billion and become the backbone of treatment in up to 60% of cancers over the next decade.

In the recurrent head and neck cancer study by Bristol-Myers Squibb, however, the median overall survival was 7.5 months for patients that responded to Opdivo. Median overall survival refers to the length of time from the start of treatment to the point where half of the patients are still alive. The other patients that received standard therapy options (cetuximab, methotrexate, and docetaxel) had a median overall survival of 5.1 months. True, there was some 20 percent of patients who had durable responses with Opdivo, but the vast majority did not.

Opdivo is a form of immunotherapy and doesn't have many of the severe side effects associated with both chemotherapy and radiation. As such, I expected to be able to continue working and not have any significant issues throughout treatment. However, releasing the brakes on the immune system can sometimes cause it to attack healthy organs and tissues in many areas of your body.

It was terrifying to think that my life expectancy could now be measured in a matter of 5-7 months. I felt like my next treatment option could be my last and therefore needed to count. And I couldn't help but think that there was a clinical trial better suited for me.

———

How to pass the time, I wondered.

While I'm not exactly an avid hiker, some of my fondest memories were from hiking the Iceline Trail in Yoho National Park and the nearby section of the Appalachian Trail with John Tedesco. In contrast to a world of smartphones and constant social media stimulation, I find that spending time hiking helps to quiet the mind and awaken all of the senses. The few times that I've done a proper hike, my body and mind always felt rejuvenated afterward. OK, my body was usually a complete wreck—but my mind was improved.

Sweet, empathetic Megan, sensing her father's zeal to hike one more time, prodded me to take her hiking on January 14th, 2017. While Rosie and I perhaps had more in common, Megan was just like Lorie—always happy to help others and put them first. Megan thought that I loved Rosie more than her as a result of our similarities, but I love them both equally.

"OK," I said. "But you'll need to get some proper boots since it could be cold and slippery at this time of the year."

We went shopping to pick up a pair of hiking boots and made plans to leave early Saturday morning. I was so excited! The prospect of sharing even a small portion of the AT together with her filled me with joy.

We left mid-morning, and it was a truly magical time. When we arrived at the Delaware Water Gap, the forest was so quiet—there wasn't a sound. There also was no breeze, so the 30-degree Fahrenheit temperature didn't feel "too" cold. Fortunately, my thoughtful wife planned and bought me a knit Cubs hat to bring along, which I did. Being vain, I hardly ever wear hats in the winter because I don't like how they mess up my hair. But boy, I was glad I did that day!

Leaving the parking lot, we navigated to the start of the trail. Given the season, the absence of vegetation made it relatively easy to follow the path. The desolate landscape, a sea of brown leaves and barren trees, was a sharp contrast to the colorful autumn scenery on my last hike.

"Look, Meg," I pointed out the white "blazes," or rectangles of white paint 2 inches wide x 6 inches high, as we walked along the trail for a few miles. I informed her that the AT is marked for daylight travel in both directions using this system of blazes that are found on trees, posts, and rocks. I chuckled to myself recalling how difficult it was to see the blazes during some portions of my hike with John. We nearly got lost on more than one occasion.

One thing we hadn't expected to find was a large rock garden with carefully balanced stones. The rocks were naturally balanced on top of one another in various positions without the use of any additional support system—some of them quite high. It was remarkable and in the middle of nowhere. *A sign from John?* I thought to myself.

With more significant respect than entering a church in the middle of a service, we navigated to the center of the garden, careful not to topple any of the stacks. Each of us placed a single rock at the top of a short stack, which was commensurate with our stone stacking skills. Next, we took turns imitating the hand position and gestures of Buddha poses and snapped some photos of each other with our phones.

Towards the end of our 5-mile loop, it began to lightly snow. It was the perfect ending to a perfect time. We paused in the middle of a bridge and took a few goofy photo selfies before heading home.

———

Knowing his expertise in immunology, I decided it was time to phone Dr. Gulley at the NIH to update him on my disease relapse and to see if he knew of any other relevant clinical trials for me. While his focus was on genitourinary cancers, such as prostate cancer, his immunotherapy research transcended into other solid tumors.

"First, I'm so sorry to hear about your condition, Michael," Dr. Gulley said during the call. "In fact, there *is* one study where I'm the principal investigator that might be ideal for you."

"Really, what is it?"

"It's a clinical trial for an investigational drug called M7824, a novel immunotherapy agent that was developed by EMD Serono, the biopharmaceutical division of Merck KGaA, Darmstadt, Germany. It is currently being studied in a Phase 1 trial for patients with advanced solid tumors, such as yours."

In addition to his role as chief of the genitourinary malignancies branch, Dr. Gulley is also director of the medical oncology service, office of the clinical director. He's an internationally recognized expert in cancer immunotherapy, and I had the honor of knowing him professionally for more than a decade, starting back when I was at Cytogen. Other key members of the NIH team included Dr. Julius Strauss, lead associate investigator for the M7824 study and fellow physician in oncology, Dr. Ravi A. Madan, clinical director of the genitourinary malignancies branch, Andrea D. Burmeister, PA, and Elizabeth Lamping RN, BSN, research nurse specialist.

Dr. Gulley explained to me that M7824 consists of a fully human monoclonal antibody that blocks PD-L1 plus a transforming growth factor beta (TGF-β)-neutralizing trap component. In simple terms, this meant that M7824 should confer all of the benefits of a checkpoint inhibitor against PD-1 or PD-L1, but with the added punch of neutralizing TGF-β, which is another crucial immune evasion target with independent yet complementary functions.

The more that I researched TGF-β, the more encouraged I became about enrolling in the M7824 clinical trial—especially given the specific profile of my disease. Based on what I had read, M7824 sounded particularly suited to work in my illness. I learned that dysregulated TGF-β signaling is a key process common to multiple HPV-related cancers.

After signing the patient consent form, I was required to pass all of the relevant tests to make sure I didn't meet any of the trial's criteria for exclusion. Most clinical trials have both entry and exclusion criteria so that they don't enroll patients with rapidly progressing disease that might not have sufficient time to respond to the drug. For example, a standard imaging procedure is done to ensure that cancer hasn't yet spread to the brain, which can result in swift, poor outcomes.

The NIH was able to rely on data and documents transferred over from MSKCC for some of the required tests.

Additional bloodwork was taken, which ended up being sufficient for me to enter the study officially.

The most significant issue arose when Dr. Gulley informed me that the sponsor of the trial, Merck KGaA, may reject me as an appropriate candidate for the study because there was a new "standard of care" option available following the recent approval of Opdivo.

Knowing that Opdivo and M7824 both had checkpoint inhibition as part of their mechanism of action, I felt that M7824 might be the better choice because it had a benefit beyond just checkpoint inhibition due to the TGF-β-neutralizing trap component.

"I looked at the M7824 materials you provided, and the agent looks quite interesting—especially in the HPV-positive setting. As such, I have great hopes for this approach. If my interpretation of the inclusion criteria is correct, I believe that I should be eligible for the study. If there's anything you can do to clarify this or revisit with Merck KGaA, I'd be extremely grateful," I informed Dr. Gulley.

"Let me see what the sponsor says based on your compelling plea," he responded.

It worked.

Dr. Gulley's next email to me confirmed that my persuasive argument was passed along to Merck KGaA and they'd agreed to include me in the study.

I was thrilled!

Participating in the study meant that I would need to commute for infusions of M7824 every other week in addition to any follow-up appointments. Getting to the NIH by train was a 2.5-hour commute from our home to Washington Union Station and then a 45-minute taxi ride to Bethesda, Maryland.

Lorie planned on accompanying me for almost every one of the trips. She found the nearby DoubleTree Hotel in Bethesda, Maryland where we could spend the night before any early morning appointments.

Before my cancer diagnosis and doing research, I had no idea that HPV is a recognized driver of six cancers, with more than 30,000 people newly diagnosed each year. Or that the HPV vaccine could prevent the majority of these cases from ever occurring. HPV cancers include cancer of the cervix, vulva, vagina, penis, or anus. HPV infection can also cause cancer in the back of the throat, including the base of the tongue and tonsils (oropharyngeal cancer).

Our family pediatrician had discussed the benefits of HPV vaccination in connection with our two daughters, so I knew about HPV and its link to cervical cancer. Naïvely, I always just assumed that the vaccines were specific to women.

The first HPV vaccine was approved by the FDA in June 2006 for use in females. It wasn't until October 2011 that the

Advisory Committee on Immunization Practices (ACIP) recommended routine use of the HPV vaccine in males aged 11 or 12 years. By that time, I was 43 years old and well-above the upper age guidance of 21 years for vaccination. Had the vaccine been available when I was much younger, it is likely that I wouldn't have developed oropharyngeal cancer.

To be an effective preventive strategy, HPV vaccination should start before sexual puberty. The CDC recommends routine HPV vaccination for girls and boys at age 11 or 12 (two doses six months apart, a 2016 revision of guidelines that previously recommended three doses). People who get vaccinated later (up to age 26 for young women and up to age 21 for young men) will need three.

According to the CDC, HPV is a prevalent virus; nearly 80 million people—about one in four—are currently infected in the United States. About 14 million people in the United States become newly infected each year.

The virus is transmitted through intimate skin-to-skin contact between mucous membranes—the moist surface layers that line organs and parts of the body that open to the outside, such as the vagina, anus, mouth, and throat. This includes having vaginal, anal, or oral sex with someone who has the virus. It may even include open-mouth kissing. In fact, it is so common that nearly all men and women get it at some point in their lives.

In most cases, HPV goes away on its own and does not cause any health problems; 9 out of 10 HPV infections go away by themselves within two years. But when HPV does not go away, persisting for years and even decades, it can cause health problems like genital warts and cancer.

Unfortunately, there is currently no simple blood test to find out a person's "HPV status." Cervical cancer screening, an essential part of a woman's routine health care, includes two types of screening tests: cytology-based screening, known as the Pap test or Pap smear, and HPV testing. Cytology-based screening is designed to detect abnormal cervical cells, including precancerous cervical lesions, as well as early cervical cancers. HPV testing is used to look for the presence of high-risk HPV types in cervical cells.

Lorie and I decided to vaccinate Rosie and Megan against HPV even before I developed cancer. After all, vaccination is widely considered one of the greatest medical achievements of modern civilization. Diseases that were commonplace less than a generation ago, such as polio, smallpox, and diphtheria, are now increasingly rare because of vaccines.

Despite the fact that vaccines are safe and usually covered by insurance, HPV vaccination still lags far behind other recommended vaccines for adolescents. According to a 2017 CDC report, only 49.5 percent of girls and 37.5 percent of boys were up to date with the recommended HPV vaccination series. Interestingly, around 80 percent of adolescents receive two other recommended vaccines (meningococcus and Tdap).

Once I went through chemoradiation treatment and suffered the associated debilitating side effects, a new segment of my "walk with purpose" became clear: Raising awareness of HPV, it's link to six cancers, and the importance of getting children vaccinated. I only wish that the HPV vaccine was available when I was a youth, as it could have prevented the cancer that's killing me.

––––––

I could hear the late British rocker Joe Cocker's version of Feelin' Alright blasting over the sound system while standing on the Trenton train platform the morning of February 1st, 2017 on my way to work in NYC. An appropriate song to start the day.

It was exactly one week ago that I'd received my first infusion of M7824 as part of the Phase 1 clinical trial at the NIH. While still very early in the process, so far I was indeed feelin' alright.

As someone who received three cycles of chemotherapy and a total radiation dose of 70 Gray over seven weeks, I can say with conviction that being treated with the immunotherapy agent was a proverbial walk in the park compared to the other therapies. In fact, if it weren't for the fact that the clinical study did not contain a placebo arm, I would seriously question whether or not I was in the active arm of the study.

For example, in contrast to chemotherapy and radiation, I hadn't experienced any of the hallmarks of traditional cancer therapy, such as nausea or fatigue, with the experimental immunotherapy agent. Of course, every drug has side effects, and checkpoint inhibitors like M7824 are associated with a unique spectrum of immune-related adverse events. These include dermatologic, gastrointestinal, hepatic, endocrine, and other less frequent inflammatory events. In some cases, these side effects can be managed with corticosteroids or diphenhydramine. Less frequently, clearly defined autoimmune systemic diseases, such as lupus, have been reported.

Having a "safe" drug is important, but for me, the real hope is that M7824 is effective in treating my recurrent disease. I read with great interest an interview with EP Vantage in January 2017, where Luciano Rossetti, Merck KGaA's head of R&D, stated that M7824 is "the most exciting clinical asset in our pipeline right now," adding that it has yielded "spectacular" early data. My hopes were high.

Following the second infusion of M7824 on February 8th, 2017, I had my periodic clinical evaluation at the NIH. At 22 days into the Phase 1 study, I was still feeling good and hadn't experienced any side effects. Blood work, vitals, etc. were all okay.

It was a quick roundtrip between home and the NIH, allowing me to be back home to spend dinner with my Valentine, wife, best friend, and birthday girl, Lorie. Before I headed out for my appointment earlier that morning, we had a few minutes to exchange greeting cards and snap a quick selfie.

Knowing that Lorie is a bit A-type and also not wanting to ruin her birthday, I waited until the next day to drop some rather significant news.

"Lorie, I would love to say that I had this all planned out, nice and neat, but I didn't, and somehow it all worked out okay in the end," I started the conversation.

"Oy!" she exclaimed. "What's going on?"

"As you know, Relmada's ongoing lawsuit has been somewhat of a distraction and drained the company's resources. It's also harder to commute to New York in addition to now commuting to the NIH in Bethesda, Maryland. So earlier this week, on Monday, I officially resigned from Relmada for personal reasons. I didn't exactly have a backup plan, but I suspected that the company might be interested in using me on a consulting basis and perhaps something could be worked out."

"You quit your job?"

"Yes, but I didn't want to tell you and ruin your birthday until I had more information. Now, I can tell you that I have a signed consulting agreement, which provides income and gives me more flexibility to work from home and not have to commute to New York daily."

"Well, thanks for not telling me until you got the consulting agreement. I think that might have finally thrown me over the edge. It sounds like you took a risky bet to be sure, but you still amaze me, Michael. I'm so proud of you, fighting so hard for us even though you're struggling with cancer and all the symptoms of your treatment."

The following week, Lorie and I took the train down to Bethesda, Maryland in advance of my third infusion with M7824. It was my first time being infused as an outpatient in the day hospital, as prior treatment required an overnight stay in the hospital for blood work, observation, etc. As with the first two infusions, everything went smoothly, with no adverse reactions during or following treatment. We caught a 9 pm train home and were in bed by 12:30 am ET.

———

The results of my routine CT imaging procedure on March 7th, 2017 were not as we had hoped. Ideally, the dozen or so tumors in my lungs would have shown signs of shrinkage, indicating that the investigational drug M7824 was having a positive effect on the cancer. Instead, several of the tumors increased in size, and a new spot even appeared in my spleen.

One of the hallmarks of immunotherapy, such as the checkpoint inhibitors, is the potential for a "delayed" response, which is not routinely seen with chemotherapy or other cytotoxic agents that tend to work quickly. Another biologic phenomenon unique to immunotherapy is the concept of "pseudoprogression," or the initial radiologic appearance of an increase in tumor burden due to inflammation that is subsequently followed by tumor regression.

The CT imaging study can't distinguish between cancer progression or inflammation as the reason for the increase in tumor size, so there was a chance that the bad results could be reversed in a month or so. It was also entirely possible, however, that the cancer wasn't responding to the treatment.

To get more details, I needed a biopsy so that one of the lung tumors could be sampled. The preliminary information from that biopsy could help distinguish between cancer progression and inflammation. Decisions regarding how to proceed would depend on that outcome.

Lorie and I had hoped to see some sign of cancer regression on the CT scan. Accordingly, many teardrops were shed before heading back home that day. The chances for a favorable outcome were diminishing, but I was persevering and intended to evaluate next steps following the biopsy results.

We headed back to the NIH on Thursday for more tests to help better guide subsequent treatment decisions. The first test in the afternoon, a CT image of my brain, would be used to rule out the spread of cancer to that particular organ. Patients with brain metastases are often excluded from clinical trials due to historically dismal survival and concerns about inadequate drug penetration through the blood-brain barrier. Fortunately, we learned the next morning that this test came back negative, so at least my cancer hadn't progressed to the brain.

We were determined to stay positive and needed a break between appointments. Taking advantage of the unseasonably warm day, we stepped outside and snapped cute selfie pictures in front of some fresh cherry blossoms. After the remaining tests were completed, we decided to go back to our room at the DoubleTree Hotel in Bethesda since it started to get cold again. It was forecast to snow the next day.

Preparing for my ultimate demise, I had recently transferred all of our home video tapes into digital formats and had them stored on my laptop computer. Lorie and I watched some of the videos to pass the time at the hotel. It was bittersweet, seeing how happy we were and all of the memories of people that had passed. Especially video of

Lorie's dad, who died unexpectedly in December 2009. We both missed him terribly.

Friday began with an image-guided biopsy of a single lung nodule to help guide between cancer progression and inflammation as the reason for the increase in size seen on the recent CT scan on the lungs. The biopsy would provide a better sense of cancer at a cellular level, which could help shed some light on whether or not treatment with M7824 was working. In my case, a core needle biopsy was performed, which is less invasive than a surgical biopsy and doesn't require general anesthesia.

Early that morning, Dr. Elliot Levy, an interventional radiologist at NIH trained in radiology and minimally invasive procedures, met with us first to discuss the process. He pulled up a cross-sectional image of my lungs, which showed several of the suspicious nodules.

One, in particular, was located in the pleural cavity— usually a thin membrane that lines the surface of the lungs and the inside of the chest wall outside the lungs. In the bottom of my left lung, however, fluid built up in the pleural cavity where one of the nodules was located.

"This nodule can be biopsied without much risk to puncturing the lung lobe," Dr. Levy explained with a confident tone. "This avoids a longer hospital stay."

Sometimes, a collapsed lung (or pneumothorax) occurs after a lung biopsy. As a precaution, a chest x-ray is taken after the procedure to check for this before sending the patient home.

After meeting with Dr. Levy, I was escorted back to the biopsy procedure room and placed on my right side on a table. I was consciously sedated with a single, intravenous dose of fentanyl that can produce excellent analgesia for 20-45 minutes, and midazolam, which has a fast-acting, short-lived sedative effect when given intravenously, achieving sedation within one to five minutes and peaking within 30 minutes. The combination produces an altered level of consciousness that still allows a patient to respond to physical stimulation and verbal commands, and to maintain an unassisted airway.

Dr. Levy worked out of sight behind me to perform the biopsy, as he inserted the needle between the ribs under my left back shoulder. I was somewhat nervous going into the procedure, but everything went well with absolutely no pain or unexpected events.

After recovery, a subsequent chest x-ray confirmed that the lungs were indeed fine after the biopsy. We left the NIH shortly after that to head back home to Pennsylvania.

The following week, Lorie and I were a bit nervous when we sat down with Dr. Strauss at the NIH to hear the biopsy results.

If the biopsy showed ample evidence of immune stimulation, an argument could be made to stay on the current drug. Under this scenario, the increase in tumor size was likely due to inflammation, and subsequent CT scans should demonstrate tumor shrinkage or regression.

However, should the biopsy results instead demonstrate increased tumor burden, then I would need to consider switching to another investigational agent or even chemotherapy to shrink the tumors.

"I'm happy to say," he began, immediately relieving our anxiety, "that based on the preliminary results it seems like M7824 might be performing as we'd hoped."

"Phew..." Lorie beamed.

"That's great to hear," I said with cautious optimism.

"Yes," Dr. Strauss went on. "I'm so happy to tell you this. At this point, I'm recommending you continue the treatment and want to schedule your next infusion here at the NIH on Tuesday. After a few more cycles of therapy, we'll take another CT scan with the hope that the recent growth was from 'pseudoprogression' rather than actual disease progression."

Knowing that I would receive my next infusion of M7824 on March 21st, 2017 as planned, Lorie and I smiled while leaving the NIH that day. But we also knew that plenty of uncertainty was still ahead.

———————

I always felt that I had a creative and artistic side, but was disappointed that my early attempts at drawing and painting never quite matched the vision in my mind. But beginning in 2011, I realized that photography allowed me to create the works of art that I envisioned.

Dreaming of one day becoming a famous photographer, I worked hard at my craft. I began advancing my knowledge of the topic by earning an associate of science degree in photography from The Art Institute of Pittsburgh, reading books, and watching instructional videos online. My work was starting to be published in numerous magazines. Unfortunately, I stopped shooting around the time that I started chemoradiation in 2016 and only managed to do a few small projects since then.

Debbie Hart of BioNJ knew of my photography interest, and we collaborated on producing a photo book commemorating the organization's 20-year anniversary back in 2013. My vision was to capture individual photographs of BioNJ's past chairmen in an environmental portrait setting.

Among others, I photographed Sol Barer at his home library, Abe Abuchowski at work, Geert Cauwenbergh holding a fine Belgium beer at a local pub in Princeton, Ken Moch at Central Park in NYC, Joe Reiser at his home wine cellar, Francois Nader in his home, and Debbie Hart standing in front of various running medals and tags, and for me, a self-portrait holding my camera.

Pleased with the results, I found myself doing more and more photography projects on the weekends. I even transformed a section of our house into a photography studio.

After my work started being published in beauty and fashion magazines, I flirted with the idea of making photography my full-time job. It was time for another one of our talks.

"How was school today? Anything exciting happen?" I asked Lorie over dinner one evening.

"My day was mostly uneventful, but the kids are already getting spring fever with the weather getting warmer," she replied. "And April is just around the corner, which marks the beginning of that long stretch of school between spring break and summer."

"Speaking of summer, I went to New Hope today to look at some spaces for rent. The town attracts a lot of visitors during the season, and I think putting a photography studio there might be a good business opportunity. The monthly rent isn't too bad, especially if I find another photographer to share the burden."

Unlike our prior talks, I knew in my heart that this one would be an uphill battle. Mainly because I was already questioning whether or not the numbers would add up.

"Oy, I don't know about doing photography full-time," said Lorie. "I know you enjoy it, and it's a fine hobby, but could you earn as much money as your prior pursuits? And what about wintertime—how many people would come to the studio then?"

It was one of the few "talks" that I lost, but she was right. Sure, if I put my mind and heart into it, I could eventually make a living through photography. Just as I had succeeded in so many other ventures. But it wasn't the right time to take on a rental studio and build a business from scratch again.

One of the important things I wanted to do before it was too late, however, was to publish a large format, high-quality, coffee table photography book of the female portraits I'd taken from 2013-2016. In reviewing my work, I curated my selection to around 200 cohesive images that I felt captured the "strength, confidence, and beauty" of women.

The images transcend fashion, fine art, and fantasy genres. Many of the photographs in the book had been published in fashion and beauty magazines such as *Elléments Magazine*, *Fuse Magazine*, *VOLO Magazine*, and *Dark Beauty Magazine* among others. Some images offered familiar settings or relatable subjects, while others incorporated slightly abstract, fantasy, or surreal elements. The subjects included professional and aspiring models, friends, celebrities, and freelance artists.

On March 25th, 2017, the hardcover and electronic version of *Strength, Confidence & Beauty* was officially launched via Blurb's self-publishing platform. I did the layout and design myself, with both hard copy and electronic PDF versions available for purchase.

It felt good to know that my photography work would be available digitally and in print long after I was gone. But I was still despondent that my lack of energy and motivation prevented me from producing much new photography work.

There was no time for self-pity, as Lorie and I reached a significant milestone with the celebration of our 25th wedding anniversary at the end of March 2017. I wasn't feeling well at the time, especially concerning appetite, so going out for a nice dinner didn't make much sense. To celebrate the silver anniversary, I wanted to get her something special and had purchased a set of Tiffany's diamond earrings.

For the majority of our decades together, Lorie always wore clip-on earrings. She had a severe allergic experience as a youth and hadn't wanted to get them pierced again. But for some reason, she decided to try again later in life, just that year in fact, and things seemed to be going okay.

After unwrapping the distinctive robin's-egg blue packaging and box, Lorie tried the earrings on right away, and they looked lovely. As I had hoped, the sparkle from the diamonds brought back a little bit of sparkle to her face. The ordinarily vivacious, upbeat, bright-eyed woman I married 25-years ago had been looking a little sad these past few months—understandably so.

Lorie's gift to me, other than 25 beautiful years together and two lovely daughters, was a framed photographic celebration of the Chicago Cubs winning the 2016 World Series. The perfect gift!

Not having a lot of energy, Lorie suggested we stay at home that evening and watch our wedding video. I recall that it seemed like a lot of money at the time, but I'm glad that we decided to videotape our wedding.

We both looked so young walking down the aisle. We had watched the tape quite a few times over the past 25-years, but I'm amazed that I never noticed something until now. Lorie smiled or laughed the *entire* day of our wedding. Even throughout the ceremony, she was grinning and giggling.

When I pointed it out to her that evening, she simply smiled.

"I was a happy bride, and it was the happiest day of my life."

Tears began to fall as we embraced on the couch watching the remainder of that truly beautiful day.

———

On Wednesday, April 12th, 2017, I started experiencing shortness of breath, coughing, and a low-grade fever which prompted a trip to the NIH with Lorie.

We arrived at the NIH that afternoon, and an x-ray confirmed that I now had a 'large' pleural effusion, which is the excessive buildup of fluid in the space between my lungs and chest cavity. Treatment involved draining the fluid from my chest cavity, either with a needle or a small tube inserted into the chest.

The pleural effusion was likely the source of my coughing, shortness of breath, and other recent symptoms. I hadn't been feeling well at all lately, but once it was drained, I was told that I should feel much better.

"You may need this treatment more than once if fluid re-collects," Dr. Levy told me before the procedure.

"OK," I replied. "I guess we'll cross that bridge another time."

Lorie waited in the lobby area as I was brought back to the operating room where Dr. Levy again worked out of sight behind me. He inserted a needle between the ribs under my left back shoulder as he did for the previous biopsy procedure, but this time connected a thin tube. I was in twilight again but watched the two glass bottles fill up quickly with the red fluid being drained from my pleural cavity.

After recovery, a subsequent chest x-ray confirmed that the lungs were fine after the procedure and we headed back up to my patient room at the NIH.

After draining the pleural effusion, I felt much better. Unfortunately, the relief didn't last long, as the fluid level in my lung had grown significantly since Wednesday. The drainage procedure had to be repeated on Good Friday.

The CT scan initially scheduled for the following week was also moved up to Friday. Lorie was quite pleased that the scan and results were being delivered on an even-numbered day. She's not superstitious, but liked even numbered days for birthdays or anything else of importance to her.

The results from the CT scan came back quickly, and they were not good.

Dr. Strauss entered the private patient room where Lorie and I were chatting with Monica Taylor, one of the clinical research nurses. Monica is terrific and always tried to stop by and say "hello" when we were there.

"First of all, how is your breathing?" Dr. Strauss inquired.

"Actually, much better. So is the coughing."

"That's good. Look, the results of the CT scan aren't what we had hoped. Several of the tumors grew since the last scan. At this point, I'm afraid it looks like this might be actual disease progression."

I was upset but tried to stay focused and practical—especially for Lorie's benefit.

"Best guess, assuming I start hospice and stop any further treatment now. How long would I live?" I asked Dr. Strauss.

"With no further therapy? My guess would be around two months."

"And if I did another round of chemotherapy?"

"Maybe 3-4 months."

"But with diminished quality of life..." I added.

Dr. Strauss nodded silently in agreement.

The news, while not overly surprising, hit us like a ton of bricks. Lorie and I asked everyone in the room for some privacy, held each other firmly, and began to sob.

Later that evening, we squeezed together in my single bed at the NIH. We mostly still cried while tightly clasping our hands together.

After what seemed like at least an hour, I cleared my throat and looked Lorie straight in the eyes.

"Honey..."

"What?"

"Listen...I don't know what's going to happen to me next or how long I'll live."

"I know, honey. You don't have to talk about it now, I understand."

"No," I said. "I want you to hear this. I want you to know that now, for the first time, I'm content. I'm at peace."

"Really?"

"Yes," I went on. "Don't get me wrong; I would love another 25 years together or even more. But my life now makes sense to me. I'm no longer the rebellious, angry child, the ambitious young man. I've proven myself, not only by having a lot of success but enduring failures and setbacks that taught me to be resilient and strong in the face of adversity."

"I know, Michael," she said softly. "And I'm so proud of you...so are the girls."

"By walking with purpose, like my father said, and by noticing, listening, appreciating the value of my bosses, colleagues, employees, and above all, you, my beautiful, wonderful wife and the two great daughters you've given me, I've finally realized the importance of empathy and true self-interest—the collective well-being of an honest effort."

Lorie was silent, listening intently, as I went on.

"I've tried to lead, to be helpful, to be a better man. Time and other people will eventually judge my success, but I'm satisfied now that, although I was never a saint or perfect human being, I've always tried to do the best I could and rarely, if ever, have I stepped away from the many, many challenges life threw at me."

I held Lorie in a close embrace for a moment, then spoke again.

"I know that you, Rosie, and Megan will face challenges going forward—especially in my absence. But I know you're strong and that you will persevere. I only hope that the children have noticed my resilience and that they too will face any future challenges head-on."

"Most of all, I look at your beauty, the glow around you, and through the large window in this NIH room, in the world we live in, the divine splendor of our life—always there if we stop to see it, to feel it around us like a radiant spirit. Now, finally, I feel that blessing...and it's enough."

A short while later, we fell asleep.

———————

Lorie and I spent Easter weekend at NIH, as I was scheduled to have an Aspira® drainage catheter surgically implanted between my ribs and into the fluid space on Monday, April 17th, 2017.

This catheter system provided a compassionate home treatment option for end-stage cancer patients like me with a malignant pleural effusion. It allowed me to drain the lung fluid buildup at home, instead of having to go to the NIH each time.

Another interventional radiologist, Dr. Venkatash Krishnasamy, or Kavi as he instructed us to call him, talked Lorie and I through the procedure in advance so we could ask questions. But he was very thorough in his explanation of the process, risks, and follow-up.

"Dr. Strauss also asked me to get another biopsy of the tumor in the pleural space if at all possible," Dr. Kavi told us, "but I'm only going to do that if I can access one of the tumors easily and not jeopardize the catheter insertion, which is our top priority at this point."

Unlike the prior drainage procedures, I was lying on my back for the catheter insertion. Dr. Kavi started inspecting the side of my left chest using ultrasound equipment.

"I think I'll be able to get the biopsy first and then complete the catheter procedure."

"Thanks, Dr. Kavi," I said amid the twilight sedation. He had a very calming bedside manner, which was much appreciated.

I was partially conscious during the procedure but didn't feel any pain before or afterward. Another liter of fluid was drained from my lung before finishing up, representing a total of four liters of fluid removed from my left lung during the week. Some of the pleural fluid would be analyzed later for clues about my disease and whether or not the experimental drug was working.

After confirming that the tunneled, long-term catheter was working correctly, Dr. Kavi taught Lorie how to perform the drainage procedure and replace the dressing. We were escorted to an empty operating room where I waited on a gurney as Lorie donned the requisite surgical gown, hair cap, facial mask, and gloves.

She looked quite professional, but it was still disconcerting that she was going to be cleaning the catheter exit site on a regular basis. Because of the location, it was awkward to handle by myself—hence the need for her to do it. While I trusted her explicitly, it made me queasy to touch the area—let alone having someone else doing it.

"You're doing a fantastic job," Dr. Kavi told Lorie as he supervised her work.

"Perhaps a new career?" I joked with her.

"Honey, I'm only able to do this for you," she replied. "I don't think I could ever be a nurse."

Dressing the wound where the catheter punctured my skin was tedious. Every day, the area needed to be cleaned and then thin layers of gauze were placed on top. Each one had a slit cut in it to make room for the clear catheter tube. Lastly, the entire area was covered in a clear, protective bandage to keep everything in place. Only a small section of tubing extended from the dressing that was periodically connected to a hand pump and bag to drain fluid as needed.

We were finally able to take the train home on Wednesday, April 19th, 2017. During the ride, I started thinking about how cancer changed our family. In particular, the negative effect cancer exerted on our family relationship, especially with the kids. In reading about the subject, I learned that a parent's cancer diagnosis impinges on a child's life by changing family routines, altering parent-child interactions, giving the child additional responsibilities, eliciting fear of potential parental death and increasing vulnerability, which add to already tricky developmental issues.[18]

Since my diagnosis, there were naturally more times when Lorie and I were stressed out or in bad moods. As a result, the girls to prefer going out with friends rather than staying home. Also, my disease became the focal point of discussion as opposed to asking Rosie and Megan about their day, what they want to eat, etc. To some extent, they were ignored.

The girls only talked about cancer when needed, but otherwise avoided any discussion or communication about the topic. When friends or relatives would ask how the family was doing or how they were doing, Rosie and Megan usually responded with "everything's fine" and tried to move on with the discussion.

I was informed by the girls' therapists not to be offended if they seem to be avoiding me—that it doesn't signal a lack of empathy. In contrast, they might love their parent so much that they cannot bear to see them decline and want to preserve the picture of the parent before getting sick. For that reason, some children stay away.

But I couldn't help but think, what if one of my procedures had gone wrong? Every time you stick a needle into the lung area, there's a risk of collapsing the lung and other potential hazards that could result in my early demise. I wondered...*how would the girls feel if they weren't there with me when I died?*

Deep in thought, I ignored the sound of Lorie's cell phone ringing until I noticed the sense of despair in her voice during the discussion.

"Okay, Dr. Dana," Lorie said hurriedly. "If you think he's that bad, please do take him to the emergency vet. Keep us posted."

"What's going on? Is Hank okay?" I asked Lorie.

Our beloved Golden Retriever, Hank, was acting more lethargic than usual during the past few days. The girls had taken him to the emergency vet the day before, but they didn't find anything wrong with him. Lorie subsequently had asked Dr. Dana Koch of HousePaws Mobile Veterinary Service to stop by the house and take a quick look at Hank.

"Dr. Dana thinks he is in terrible shape and needs to go back to the emergency vet right away."

"Oh no."

"Megan is going with her, and they are taking him over there now."

Anyone who knows our family will attest to the fact that we are insane animal lovers. But for me, Hank held an extraordinary place in my heart. Aside from being the only other male in our house, he brought a ton of laughter and joy into our lives since his arrival in February 2008. Especially when I needed it most during my existential crisis later that same year.

A short while later, Lorie's cell phone rang again.

"Hello?"

"Lorie, it's Dr. Jennifer Adler from the Center for Animal Referral and Emergency Services."

"How is Hank?"

"I'm afraid I have some awful news," Dr. Adler replied. "There is a bacterial infection ravaging his kidneys and heart. Unfortunately, there is nothing we can do."

"Oh, no! Can you at least keep him comfortable for a little while? We're on the train heading home and will try to get there as fast as possible. We'd like to say goodbye before..."

"Absolutely, and I'm sorry—I know your life has been difficult enough lately," Dr. Adler interjected as Lorie struggled to speak, choking back tears.

After arriving at the Trenton, New Jersey train station, we drove quickly home to get Rosie and Megan and then raced over to the Center for Animal Referral and Emergency Services (CARES). Upon arrival, a nurse ushered us to a dimly lit, private grieving room. *Were we too late?* I wondered.

A few minutes later, the back door opened and a solemn Dr. Adler appeared. Hank was lying on a gurney as she wheeled him into the room. He was motionless and seemed to be comfortable. As soon as he saw our family, his soulful eyes brightened—he knew he wasn't alone and that we were all there by his side. We took turns hugging him and saying goodbye as Dr. Adler administered the drugs that sent him on a long, peaceful slumber. He would have been ten years old later that year.

What's the old proverb? "It never rains, but it pours." The trouble with clichés is that they're usually true.

———————

The next day, just before Lorie was about to change the dressing for my chest tube, Dr. Strauss called my cell phone.

"I wanted to provide an update following our discussion last Friday afternoon, is now a good time?" he asked.

"Yes, please. Go ahead," I replied, placing the phone on speaker so that Lorie could hear as well.

"I was informed that the pathology from your pleural fluid revealed no evidence of cancer cells but only evidence of chronic inflammation. While it's possible that the pleural effusion is due to cancer and cancer cells may have been missed in the analysis, I think it is also a possibility that the pleural effusion is related to inflammation from the M7824 treatment."

"Isn't that good news?" I asked. "Couldn't it mean that the tumor growth on the latest scan could still be pseudoprogression?"

"Yes," he replied. "In fact, one of my colleagues had a patient with lung cancer just this last week, who was responding to the same treatment you received and also developed a pleural effusion thought to be related to inflammation."

"So, what does this all mean?" Lorie asked.

"Well, although it's standard practice to assume increasing lesions at two consecutive scans are in fact disease progression, we had at least one case of a patient receiving this treatment who had pseudoprogression for several months before his lesions began to shrink."

"What about the biopsy of the tumor?" I asked.

"The recent biopsy also showed an increase in immune cells compared to the last biopsy, which further supports that the drug is working. I guess what I'm saying is that in contrast to the information we had available to us last week, I'm now leaning more towards keeping you on M7824 or putting you on another immunotherapy trial as opposed to chemotherapy to see if we can help the body's immune system take over the disease."

"So, what would be the next steps?"

"In a couple of weeks, I'd like to do another CT scan to look at the tumors. We have you on a low dose steroid to help sculpt the inflammatory response and reduce the amount of fluid being produced in your left lung. However, the steroids could also impact the inflammation surrounding the other tumors, such as those in your right lung. If we see any signs of stabilization or even regression on the next CT scan in those areas, it would be one more piece of evidence that what we see regarding growth is pseudoprogression as opposed to disease progression."

After the call, Lorie continued attending to my chest tube. She put on rubber gloves, carefully removed the clear bandage and then the gauze. Next, Lorie would clean the area with alcohol wipes. I got weirded out each time she touched the tubing to move and clean around it, but she was always gentle. Finally, she would replace the gauze and bandage before I connected the catheter to a bag for drainage.

The Aspira drainage system had dramatically improved the pleural effusion. My left lung, which was previously two-thirds blocked from the fluid, was now close to normal following drainage.

Also, the prescribed steroid (prednisone) helped "sculpt" the inflammatory response and kept the fluid from building up so quickly in my lung. Whereas I was previously emptying 100 mL or more on a daily basis, now I was now only draining 15-20 mL every other day or so.

With the pleural effusion effectively managed, attention returned to whether or not to resume treatment with M7824. My last infusion of M7824 was several weeks ago.

Following another CT scan and constructive discussion with the NIH team, we concluded that there is a tug-of-war occurring between cancer and my body's immune system. The hope is that eventually M7824 will tip the scale in favor of my body's immune system and control the cancer.

Accordingly, the decision was made to keep moving forward with M7824. I was scheduled to receive an infusion on Tuesday, May 16, 2017. The pleural effusion would be monitored closely and managed via the catheter and steroids. A repeat CT scan would be done in a month or so to reassess the situation.

While this latest development was a bit more encouraging, we were still hoping for the best and prepared for the worst. Figuring that I had only a few months left to live, it was time to start the grim task of getting my affairs in order.

Our family and friends were in Illinois, but the East Coast was now our home. Lorie and I discussed whether to have my body buried in Illinois or Pennsylvania. In the end, we went with the nearby Newtown Cemetery Association, a local, non-denominational cemetery, and arranged a meeting to pick out plots. Sadly, it was the first and only real estate purchase we made that didn't require a mortgage.

"We have a lot of spots available, so it depends on your preference—facing east or west, even or odd number lots, things like that," superintendent Eric Johnson started off.

"I guess I'd rather everyone was facing west during the ceremony," I offered after surveying the location. "Looking towards the chapel building...I don't know; it just seems more serene."

"I agree," Lorie said.

"Okay then, let's head over to the other side," Eric said as he started walking, carrying the map of available plots.

We strolled over, noticing the variations in headstones. Some had photographs of the deceased embedded in the stone; others had detailed, etched drawings. Personally, I preferred the simple, understated headstones.

Lorie and I held hands walking to lot #14. Knowing her penchant for even numbers, it seemed like as good a choice as any. There we stood, deep in thought about the prospects that in the not-so-distant future we would be back here, each of us under slightly different circumstances. It was quite surreal.

I looked down at the grassy spot where I would eventually be buried, admiring the blooming cherry trees and beauty of the location. For some reason, I had a sense of relief knowing where I would be at rest, and most importantly that Lorie and I would eventually be in the same location.

When we returned to Eric's office, we discussed the option of buying two additional plots for Rosie and Megan. He informed us that the plots could be sold or transferred, so if the kids didn't ultimately want to use them, they didn't have to. We wanted to give them at least the option of being buried right next to us and opted to get the additional space.

Feeling as though we were tying up some of the loose ends helped me feel better that my family would eventually be okay, giving me further peace of mind. Lorie took a leave of absence from work for the rest of the school year so we could focus on enjoying the remainder of our time together.

It is difficult to stay upbeat and positive in the face of a terminal cancer diagnosis. But keeping busy and trying new things can help.

I started acupuncture and sound therapy with Sharon Czebotar, a Nationally Board Certified, Licensed Acupuncturist and Oriental Medicine Practitioner. I was skeptical about acupuncture until being offered the service while inpatient at the NIH. I found the therapy helped with appetite, neuropathy, and more, which convinced me to search out a local expert. Sharon also recommended a separate class on transcendental meditation, which I started along with Rosie the following weekend.

Beyond these activities, whenever Lorie or I start getting a little depressed or down, she redirects the conversation to happier topics—and quickly rattles off the phrase "puppies, kittens, rainbows, and unicorns." Of the four options, I found puppies the easiest to embrace—and potentially acquire. Besides, we had enough cats already.

The recent passing of Hank weighed heavily on my shoulders, so we began to consider a new addition to the

Becker zoo. We started with local animal shelters but had trouble finding a good match for us.

There was no replacing Hank, but the house seemed empty without a Golden Retriever. To scratch that itch, we decided to visit the breeder where we initially got Hank to play with some puppies. We were setting ourselves up for failure, as one does not merely "window shop" for puppies.

Upon arrival, we parked the car and were greeted by a young Golden named Spanky. His resemblance to Hank was uncanny, and we spent some time playing with him in the open lot before spotting Amy, the breeder.

She informed us that Spanky was the father of a 4-week old litter of 11 puppies that we could play with and see. More importantly, we learned that Spanky and Hank were blood relatives. Clearly, we were getting a puppy.

But puppies shouldn't be separated from their mother until they are at least 8-weeks old. Over the next month, we visited the puppies as they grew. Each time brought us tremendous joy. Especially when all eleven pups would rush to greet us from their fenced play area—ears flopping, tails wagging, and bodies tumbling. And during each visit, Spanky greeted us at the car to play.

We returned during the first week of June to select one of only four males out of the litter. The largest puppy from the litter was just irresistible. We named him Humphrey and brought him home.

With everything going on in our lives, along with an uncertain future, a puppy was the last thing that our family needed. My fatigue and overall health condition meant that Lorie would be taking on the lion's share of the additional work. And raising a puppy is a lot of work!

But Humphrey was precisely what I needed. Even more so than I realized at the time. He provided me with comfort, comic relief, and a distraction from stress. Most importantly, he offered a sense of companionship that helped combat feelings of isolation when Lorie and the girls weren't around.

One of the hallmarks of Golden Retrievers is their endearing, silly streak. In fact, according to the American Kennel Club, Goldens "take a joyous and playful approach to life and maintain this puppyish behavior into adulthood." Humphrey is no exception; he makes us laugh constantly.

———

Although we made many trips to Bethesda, Maryland for my NIH appointments, we didn't explore the city or many of the local establishments. On July 11th, 2017, Lorie and I decided to grab an early dinner in the town at a nice restaurant recommended to us. It was enjoyable to venture out and try something new.

We sat down, and I immediately focused on the cheese appetizer selection and ordered three different types. Halfway through the appetizer, however, my cell phone rang. It was Dr. Strauss from the NIH.

I could tell from his initial line of questioning (are you still at the NIH, where are you now, are you alone, etc.) that bad news would shortly follow. Sure enough, the prior day's CT scan revealed a deep vein thrombosis (DVT) on the left side of my pelvis, and Dr. Strauss requested that we promptly return to NIH to start treatment with a blood thinner. With that news, we paid our restaurant bill, left our dinners behind, and rushed to get back to the NIH.

Both Dr. Gulley and Dr. Strauss met us back at the day hospital, and we went to an empty treatment room to talk in private. Unfortunately, the blood clot was merely a sideshow for the bigger news, which was that several tumors increased in size from the prior scan taken 6-weeks ago. For the first time, my outlook was black & white: cancer was winning the tug-of-war with my body's immune system. Receiving further treatment with the experimental agent M7824 would be hard to justify, so was taken off the clinical study. More aggressive treatment, such as chemotherapy, appeared to be the recommended next step.

After a brief tutorial on self-injecting Lovenox® (enoxaparin) twice daily, we returned to the hotel and planned on meeting early the next morning to review the CT scans and have further discussion. The mood was somber, and neither one of us slept very well.

The next morning, we arrived at NIH, one of only two places in the world to have advanced imaging technology that was truly fascinating and dramatically improves the ability to visualize and follow specific tumors over time. We were engrossed in discussion with Dr. Gulley about the various images displayed on three monitor screens when Lorie's cell phone rang. Caller ID showed it was Rosie.

The first few calls were easy to dismiss since we were in an important meeting. But then came a simple text message from Rosie—"emergency." Driving home from class, Rosie was involved in a car accident. All of the airbags deployed and the car was totaled. She was taken to the local hospital for x-rays, but nothing was broken, and she was later released without incident.

Immediately, my mind darted from my mortality being visualized on the computer screens to how Rosie's accident could have been far, far worse – perhaps even fatal. I'm not sure exactly how I would have reacted to that news on top of my disease update, but I do know it would pale in comparison to my situation.

On more than one occasion, Lorie and I have uttered the words "it could always be worse." Lately, it has been harder and harder to make that statement. However, with Rosie mostly unharmed in what could have been disastrous, today definitely could have been worse.

With no infusion of M7824 warranted following the CT scan results, we headed home to be with Rosie.

Chapter Ten
Third Time's a Charm?

———

The distinction between quality and quantity of life isn't subtle. Going through chemotherapy again, even without radiation this time, would be anything but fun. The prospect of experiencing fatigue, nausea, appetite changes, increased susceptibility to infection, and more in exchange for perhaps gaining a few extra months of life didn't seem like a fair trade.

Forgoing further treatment while being made comfortable through hospice care seemed like a nicer option. However, I didn't stop to think about the fact that there are better and worse ways to die. Or, that no one knows precisely when or how they will pass. My overly simplistic view was that cancer would continue to grow, eventually disrupting a critical organ or function, and that would be the end. Hopefully, this would occur in the middle of a deep slumber one night, and I wouldn't wake the next day. Quick and easy, or so I hoped.

Thankfully, a follow-up conversation with Dr. Strauss at the NIH helped change my perspective. He asked me to reconsider chemotherapy as a next step, stating it could buy more time than just a few months. And if the side-effects were intolerable, Dr. Strauss reminded me that I could always discontinue treatment at any time. Even one cycle of chemotherapy could help shrink the tumors and lead to potentially better outcomes with future immunotherapy approaches. Exploring the vast array of possibilities, it was also clear that the odds of a quick and easy demise were remote.

Case in point, I had been on a blood thinner for just under one week, when I noticed that the daily drainage from my chest tube looked much more like blood than the usual straw color. Equally disconcerting, the volume of fluid was higher than usual.

The only new variable—the blood thinner—likely played a role. While discontinuing it could help reverse the bleeding, I would be left with an untreated blood clot that could cause major problems if it moved from its current location.

Quite the problem and not one to take lightly. After a brief conversation with the physician-on-call at MSKCC, Lorie drove us to New York City on Sunday evening, July 16th, 2017, to the urgent care facility. I already had an appointment scheduled with my medical oncologist, Dr. Pfister, for Tuesday to discuss possible next-steps for treatment, including chemotherapy.

We arrived after midnight, and the urgent care team promptly assessed my condition. Blood work was drawn along with ordering a chest x-ray and CT scan. Looking at the chest x-ray results, I could tell that the pleural effusion in my left lung had grown quite large. This shouldn't be the case, as I drained it daily.

Stopping any internal bleeding was more important than addressing the blood clot—although both issues required immediate attention. Use of the blood thinner was discontinued and the medical staff considered how to best access and drain a large amount of fluid trapped in my left lung. The impact of the fluid was significant, as I was short of breath walking even short distances. My cough was also worse and caused me to feel light-headed and dizzy.

On Monday, a vacuum-like device was connected to my chest tube, and the fluid gradually turned to a healthier yellowish color. Next, I was put back on the blood thinner while continually monitoring the fluid output through the transparent tube—fearful that the color would change back to blood red. Fortunately, the color remained the same.

The next day, Lorie and I spoke with Dr. Pfister about options for my third line of therapy, one of which included a cocktail of drugs—two chemotherapies along with a biologic agent. This involved 5-fluorouracil (5-FU), cisplatin or carboplatin, and the monoclonal antibody Erbitux® (cetuximab). Initially, I discounted this option because 5-FU-based regimens can be associated with significant toxicities. One of the many nasty side effects from 5-FU is palmar-plantar erythrodysesthesia, also known as hand-foot syndrome (HFS). There are currently no treatments or preventions for HFS, which is characterized by tingling in the palms, fingers, and soles of feet and by erythema, which may progress to burning pain with dryness, cracking, peeling, ulceration, and more. Coincidentally, I learned a lot about HFS while serving as CEO of VioQuest Pharmaceuticals. The company was developing a topical formulation to prevent HFS potentially.

Based in part on my concern, Dr. Pfister suggested replacing 5-FU with weekly paclitaxel, resulting in a chemotherapy regimen known as PCC (paclitaxel, carboplatin, and cetuximab) that has been found to be efficacious and well-tolerated in patients when used as induction chemotherapy. 5-FU and paclitaxel can be viewed as somewhat interchangeable, but paclitaxel offers a more favorable toxicity profile.

In contrast to the two chemotherapeutics, Erbitux is an older biologic agent. It is a "chimeric" monoclonal antibody, which is made by joining antibody genes from two different species; in this case human and mouse. Newer monoclonal antibodies are often fully human, which reduces the risk of a reaction to foreign antibodies from a non-human animal.

Erbitux targets and binds to epidermal growth factor receptors (EGFR) that are found on the surface of many healthy cells and cancer cells. Doing so stops the cell from continuing the signaling pathway that promotes cell division and growth, effectively stopping the cancer by preventing the cancerous cells from growing and multiplying. Unfortunately, normal skin cells also have a lot of EGFR, so drugs that target or block EGFR can negatively affect skin cells.

I knew about Erbitux and expressed my reservations about the potential for severe skin toxicities including skin rash, skin dryness, pruritus, paronychia, hair abnormality, and mucositis. As a result, Dr. Pfister suggested forgoing Erbitux and moving forward with just the two chemotherapeutics. His rationale was that Erbitux could always be utilized later if needed.

Under the dual chemotherapy regimen, one cycle of treatment is comprised of four weeks. During week one, two different chemotherapeutics (carboplatin and paclitaxel) are given along with the requisite premedication (steroid, anti-nausea meds, and an antihistamine). But during both the second and third weeks of a cycle, I receive only one chemotherapeutic (paclitaxel) and the same premeds. Week four is a holiday/break, with no scheduled treatment that helps provide recovery time for blood counts and other markers. Then the four-week cycle repeats.

Much to my surprise, I was able to start treatment with the next day, July 18th, 2017, while still in the hospital. I never thought I'd be happy to say the phrase "I'm back on chemotherapy." But there I was, continuing the fight.

Why? Because Lorie slept at a hotel on our second night in NYC to get some much-needed rest. My mind went drifting down memory lane as I sat alone in the patient room at MSKCC. I thought about all the good times we shared, the family we raised, and how much we love each other. I wept and wept. Suddenly, I realized that if chemotherapy could give me even just one more day with her, it would be worth the drug's side effects. And yes, there is still the hope of doing better and living longer than expected. The chances are remote, but not zero.

The purpose of the chemotherapy treatment is palliative—to keep the tumors in my lungs and other organs from growing to a point where they cause pain, breathing difficulty, and other issues. It is different from care to cure your illness, called curative treatment.

When treatment is palliative, some patients may feel uncomfortable asking their doctor, "How long do you think I have to live?" The truth is that this question is often awkward for doctors too. Nonetheless, it is a question on the mind of many terminal cancer patients—including me.

Every patient is different, and a statistical prognosis is just an estimate, not a firm prediction. For example, last summer I was in terrible shape (two chest tubes, progressive disease, blood clot and bleeding issues, rapid heart rate requiring a stay in the ICU, etc.). The prognosis at that time was grim, and I wasn't expected to live more than a few months.

Fortunately, my situation improved dramatically since then.

———

The following Sunday, Lorie and I drove to New York City for another visit to MSKCC's urgent care facility. Drainage from my chest tube once again changed from amber to the color of a fine Cabernet wine, signaling that bleeding had resumed. More alarming was the accompanying shortness of breath and increased coughing. I was out of breath even from walking a short distance to go to the bathroom.

We arrived at MSKCC around mid-morning and, following a brief review of recent events, had a chest x-ray taken to get a quick read on the situation. The resulting images showed a complete "white-out" of my left lung, which indicated that fluid had essentially filled the entire space. Usually, the lungs look transparent or black on an x-ray due to air in the lungs.

The fact that I had only one viable lung explained the shortness of breath and coughing. What the x-ray couldn't reveal was the composition of the fluid (serous fluid, blood, etc.) or its source. For more information, a CT scan was required and scheduled. Unfortunately, weekends at any hospital can be hectic, and my CT scan didn't take place until close to midnight. I was admitted.

Monday morning, we had the pleasure of meeting again with surgeon Dr. Bernard Park, deputy chief of clinical affairs, thoracic service at MSKCC. In December 2016, Dr. Park had successfully performed a bronchoscopy procedure to biopsy a suspicious lymph node near my airway. We knew that we were in good hands.

"For whatever reason, the catheter in your left lung isn't fully draining the fluid—especially towards the top section of your lung," Dr. Park started. "That fluid needs to be drained to alleviate your shortness of breath and coughing."

"How do we best accomplish this?" I asked.

"My preference would be a short-term solution where we temporarily insert a plastic tube straight through the front of your chest into the top section of the lung to manually extract the fluid. This would require a brief stay in the hospital while the tube was present and it would be removed before going home."

"Any other options, Dr. Park?" Lorie inquired.

"A longer-term solution would be to place a second catheter that could be accessed whenever needed at home to extract fluid from the top section of the lung. But in either case, a potential pitfall is that the fluid in the upper section of the lung may be trapped in pockets by fibrotic scar tissue or tumor, preventing effective drainage."

Dr. George Getrajdman, an interventional radiologist at MSKCC, proposed a step-wise procedure. First, he would try to extract the fluid near the top of the left lung using a syringe to see "if" anything could be extracted. If so, he could confidently proceed with placement of a second catheter (Option A) or the fluid could simply be drained with the syringe to see if that provided symptomatic relief before moving forward with a more permanent catheter placement (Option B). Placing a temporary plastic tube was also a consideration (Option C), with the downside being that fluid could accumulate again in the future and require another procedure. If no fluid could be extracted with a syringe, then the space was being occupied by something more substantial (fibrotic scar tissue or tumor mass), and a catheter would be pointless. Ultimately, I decided to proceed with Option A.

Requiring more urgent resolution, however, was the recently discovered blood clot in my iliac vein near the pelvis and its potential to detach and cause a pulmonary embolism (PE)—a condition in which one or more arteries in the lungs become blocked by a blood clot, which could stop blood flow to the lung. With essentially only one lung currently functioning, a PE in my remaining viable lung would likely be fatal. Hence the sense of urgency.

Due to the recurrence of blood in the drainage from my original chest tube, we reached the point where taking anticoagulant medication was no longer viable and was discontinued. The only alternative was the placement of an inferior vena cava (IVC) filter device designed to trap/prevent my blot clot from traveling from the largest vein in the body, the inferior vena cava, to the lungs or heart.

To insert an IVC filter, I was given medication to help relax and a local anesthetic to numb the area of insertion. Implanting the IVC filter was Dr. Getrajdman, who inserted a catheter through a small incision in my neck. Using X-rays images to guide the procedure, he advanced the IVC filter through the catheter and into the inferior vena cava. Once the IVC filter was in place, he removed the catheter and put a small bandage on the insertion site.

Fortunately, Dr. Getrajdman was also able to deal with the left lung issue during the same procedure. Approximately 1.5 liters of fluid was successfully acquired from the top portion of the lung, so he proceeded with the placement of a second catheter as planned. Both procedures took about 1.5 hours in total to complete. Afterward, an x-ray confirmed that the top portion of the lung was free of fluid.

My breathing improved immediately following the procedure, and I felt just fine with all of the pain medication. However, waking up Tuesday morning I felt like I'd been hit by a truck. There was a fair amount of pain at both the incision on my neck from the IVC filter insertion and the newly placed catheter site. As the day progressed, the pain diminished, and I started feeling much better.

By late afternoon, Lorie and I were trained on using the "new" PleurX catheter and then proceeded with draining fluid from both the top and bottom catheters. The top PleurX catheter rapidly removed 500 cubic centimeters of fluid, which looked far less bloody than what had previously been extracted from the bottom. We were only able to drain 200 cubic centimeters of fluid from the prior Aspira catheter, which was still bloody and thicker. It's speculated that the fluid from the bottom was left over from before and there was no active bleeding, which would be confirmed by monitoring my hemoglobin levels.

With the IVC filter in place and the ability to drain both top/bottom fluid from my left lung, I was able to proceed with my second dose of chemotherapy while in the hospital. By Wednesday, subsequent chest x-rays showed a further reduction in fluid from my left lung, and I was released from the hospital the following day. I was anxious to get home and see how big our new puppy Humphrey had grown in the short time we'd been away.

On Tuesday, August 1st, 2017, I received my third dose of chemotherapy. Everything went well, and the next day I was feeling good. As an added plus, I was looking forward to having Dad, Linda, Brandy and her family in town for the weekend. Life seemed okay at the moment.

In the back of my mind, I knew that I likely hadn't reached the nadir, or lowest point, in my blood counts from the prior chemotherapy. As such, there was a possibility that I might not be feeling 100 percent for my visitors by the weekend.

Sure enough, by Wednesday evening I started running a mild temperature. No big deal—it was below the cutoff of 100.4 degrees Fahrenheit for an "official" temperature. On Thursday, I wasn't feeling energetic and napped most of the day. Then the real fun started.

My temperature became official Thursday evening, and the physician-on-call at MSKCC recommended that I come to urgent care to get things checked out. So, Lorie and I made the drive to New York City for the third visit to urgent care within the past three weeks! We debated taking the train as opposed to driving, which would have been faster.

By the time we arrived at MSKCC, my temperature was above 102 degrees Fahrenheit, and I felt the familiar muscle aches and general fatigue that I associated with influenza. Coincidentally, it was the diagnosis of influenza during my first week of chemoradiation in early 2016 that resulted in my first trip to MSKCC's urgent care facility.

Flu season doesn't usually begin until October, so this time the concern was a bacterial infection. With my white blood cell counts negatively impacted by chemotherapy, it was possible that my body couldn't fight off an infection in one of my chest tubes or another location.

I was triaged with the usual battery of blood tests and a chest x-ray before being placed in an exam room. Urgent care was very crowded that evening. I was just happy to have a bed and looked forward to resting horizontally for a while.

I sat on the bed, preparing to relax and lay down.

"Honey, what's wrong?!" Lorie asked as I clutched my chest from a sudden, stabbing pain.

"I'm not sure, but my chest really hurts," I replied, grimacing from the discomfort.

Lorie could tell from the expression on my face this was no ordinary situation.

"I need immediate help," Lorie said after pressing the emergency call button. "My husband is having chest pain."

A nurse arrived without delay to assess the situation. As she connected various cables to my body, I felt my heart racing, and we were shocked to see my pulse rate appear on the computer monitor. It was 225. Normally, the heart beats about 60 to 100 times per a minute. But in tachycardia, the heart beats faster than normal while at rest.

The episode ended within a minute or so, but tachycardia can disrupt healthy heart function and lead to severe complications, including heart failure, stroke, and sudden cardiac arrest or death. Defibrillator adhesive patches were applied outside of my chest wall, which could be used if needed to provide a brief electric shock to reset the heart rhythm back to its normal, regular pattern.

My heart wasn't the only thing racing. The medical team rushed to place a crash cart outside my door, and a sense of urgency filled the room. The contents of a crash cart vary, but typically contain the tools and drugs needed to treat a person in or near cardiac arrest. Having seen enough television hospital dramas, I was sure that the end was near.

Fortunately, no further cardiac events occurred, and I was admitted to MSKCC's intensive care unit (ICU), where seriously ill patients are cared for by specially trained staff. While I never had the misfortune to be admitted to an ICU in the past, I was amazed by both the medical staff and technology used to monitor my condition and knew I was in excellent hands. Nevertheless, and despite going against hospital policy, Lorie wasn't leaving my side and insisted on staying the night with me in the ICU.

My wife is one of the most loving and compassionate people I know. As a school teacher, she has a deep sense of care and genuine concern for others. She is very sweet—even earning the nickname Mary Poppins at work. That is until you mess with someone she loves. Doing so transforms this kind, gentle person into "mama bear"—a terrifying force to be reckoned with.

"How did you get them to let you stay the night?" I asked.

"Nobody messes with mama bear," Lorie replied in a protective tone.

"Oh, I see. But no bloodshed or incriminating bruises this time, right?" I replied jokingly with a wink of the eye.

"You can still make me laugh."

I was placed on an antibiotic and medication to stabilize my heart rate while the team worked to determine the source of the tachycardia and whether or not my episode had caused any damage to my heart. Preliminary assessments ranged from one of my tumors or chest tubes rubbing up against the sensitive tissue surrounding the heart to low electrolyte levels, which are essential minerals in your body that have an electric charge. Maintaining the right balance of electrolytes is critical for your body's blood chemistry, muscle action, and other processes.

On Friday, my temperature returned to normal, and there were no further cardiac events. Still, I couldn't help but feel that perhaps it was time to contact hospice and let cancer take its course. I had faced my share of obstacles since being diagnosed with cancer in late 2015, and three recent trips to the hospital resulted in further erosion of my quality of life with two chest tubes, being back on chemotherapy and its side effects, and now the prospect of potential cardiac issues. Lorie and I briefly discussed the topic of hospice, but she rightfully pointed out that such a decision shouldn't be made while sitting in the ICU.

Later that afternoon, I shared my thoughts about hospice with a nurse while he assisted me with walking a few laps around the ICU floor. Much to my surprise, he shared with me that about 11-years ago he underwent a bone marrow transplant at MSKCC and how it caused him to pursue a career in medicine. He quickly discounted my outlook on hospice, stating that I was young, up-and-walking, and seemed otherwise quite capable of enjoying further quality time with my family.

Rosie and Megan traveled by train to NYC so that they could visit me. Sitting upright in my bed after my walk, I smiled at the sight of them through the massive glass wall that faced the hallway. I felt like an animal on display at the zoo. However, with the push of a button, the special electrochromic glass wall could turn from clear to opaque and back again—offering privacy on demand.

Before the girls came into the room, Lorie offered to bring me some macaroni and cheese for dinner, and they all left for a short while. Unintendedly, by the time they returned with food the visiting hours were over and they weren't allowed to come back in. Instead, they dropped off my meal, and all stayed overnight at a nearby hotel thanks to the generosity of my father and Linda. Being in the ICU wasn't conducive to their planned visit that weekend, which unfortunately got canceled.

Early the next morning, Lorie returned to the ICU alone since the girls liked to sleep late. Sitting bedside, she was holding my hand when we noticed a tall shadow through the opaque glass wall. The figure appeared to be engaged in a conversation with one of the nurses stationed outside of my room.

WHOOSH! The electrochromic glass wall suddenly became transparent, revealing Dr. Pfister.

"I've been following what happened and thought I'd stop by since I had a meeting in the area this morning," he said through the doorway.

"What a surprise! That's very nice of you," Lorie and I replied in unison.

"I wanted to let the nurse know that your blood counts may be on the decline from the prior dose of chemotherapy so that they weren't surprised. I also see that Dr. Sanjay Chawla is checking up on you—he's an excellent intensive care specialist, so you're in great hands."

I was released from the ICU to a regular room very late that evening. The medical staff informed me that I'd be in the hospital for at least another day or two because the source of my fever still hadn't been identified. With the temperature gone, it appeared that the antibiotics were successful in treating the infection. But without knowing the source or bacterial strain—effective treatment can be challenging.

By Saturday afternoon, Lorie, Rosie, and Megan were able to visit longer since I was now out of the ICU and in a regular room. Seeing people in the hospital isn't tops on most teen's lists of favorite activities, but it meant so much having them there.

My recent hospitalization was the longest and most volatile, resembling that of a roller coaster ride at an amusement park. What started with a fever prompting our arrival at MSKCC's urgent care facility last Thursday evening ended up escalating to a brief stay in the ICU.

The isolated cardiac event was managed by medication (metoprolol) and didn't reappear. However, despite numerous blood cultures, chest x-rays, CT scans, and other diagnostics, the cause of my fever—the original reason for my hospital visit—remained a mystery.

After an infectious disease consult, bacterial infection was ruled out as the likely source of the fever, and I was taken off the broad-spectrum antibiotics that were being delivered via intravenous infusion. Some of the cultures take time to process, so there was always a chance that something could materialize in the coming days.

One silver lining amidst the tight turns, steep slopes, and inversions on my roller coaster ride was the fact that my left lung appeared much improved in terms of fluid accumulation. This coincided with almost zero drainage from my two chest tubes over the past week or so.

The medical team determined that removing both of my chest tubes was in my best interest. They weren't serving any functional purpose, and there is always a risk of infection by having two foreign objects in the body.

Insertion of the two chest tubes, one while at the NIH and the other at MSKCC, were both done under twilight anesthesia. I was awake but sedated. This was accomplished via administration of a concoction of agents including a benzodiazepine (midazolam) and the narcotic fentanyl. For both procedures, I had little discomfort.

Naturally, I just assumed that removal of the chest tubes would also be done under twilight anesthesia. Much to my chagrin, I was informed that the extraction procedure is typically done bedside in the hospital without anesthesia. Two medical professionals from interventional radiology arrived at my room at MSKCC and provided a reasonable explanation for the lack of lidocaine or other local anesthesia. They stated that the injections would hurt more than the extraction since several would be needed to cover the entire area. There was also a risk that the chest tubes could be punctured via the needles.

"I don't think this bedside process sounds right," Lorie said to me in private. "I'm going to step out and call Dr. Kavi's cell phone and ask how the NIH usually handles catheter removal. At the very least, I'm also going to ask one of the nurses to at least give you a dose of oxycodone before doing anything."

Mama bear was back in action.

Ever since their initial placement, I've been anxious when anyone cleans or touches the plastic tubes that protrude from the front of my left chest. Something was unnerving about seeing plumbing sticking out from my body. It seemed better suited on a Borg, a fictional alien group that appeared in the Star Trek franchise.

Lorie stepped back into the room after being unable to reach Dr. Kavi. One of the nurses did bring me some pain medication, although there wasn't enough time for it to kick in.

I was quite apprehensive when one of the medical professionals wrapped the end of the first tube around her hand once or maybe twice. Then, she proceeded to yank it as if she was pulling the cord to start a lawnmower. To be fair, the pain wasn't terrible, and this was one of those situations where speed was better than slowly dragging it out. Nonetheless, I was shocked by the experience and now had an idea what extraction of the second tube would be like.

The first tube was smooth by comparison, as it was only placed a short while ago. The second extraction was more difficult since that tube was in place for 4-months and had grown quite attached to me. The first attempt at pulling yielded little, if any, movement from the tube. Fortunately, the second try was successful. I was now completely free of chest tubes. The tips of both tubes were cut and sent to be cultured in case either was the source of infection that was causing my fevers.

There were plenty of other possibilities to explain my fevers, including the tumors, blood clots, and others. For now, the plan was to return home and carefully monitor my temperature—hoping that it continued responding to acetaminophen. If not, we'd be back at the hospital.

Given the current situation, Dr. Pfister understandably held back on that week's cycle of chemotherapy to be safe. Encouragingly, the CT scan used to look for pneumonia and other potential reasons for the fever provided a sneak peek of how the tumors responded to my first three weeks of chemotherapy. Almost all of the tumors showed decreases in size! This was better than having the tumors grow or stay the same size, although it didn't change the "terminal" nature of my disease.

Bacterial cultures from the tips of two chest tubes that were recently removed revealed the growth of a Pseudomonas organism on one of them. These are relatively common pathogens involved in infections acquired in a hospital setting. Whether or not this was the source of my fevers, I was prescribed an antibiotic (levofloxacin, 500mg daily) since pseudomonas can lead to other nasty conditions.

I continued running a fever for a few days after starting the antibiotic but was free of fever for the 48-hours leading up to my next scheduled round of chemotherapy. Aside from the mystery fever, my blood counts were excellent throughout the three weeks of chemotherapy. Dr. Pfister supported resuming treatment.

The consensus was that my rapid heartbeat was caused by a perfect storm consisting of a high fever, low electrolytes, and possible bacterial infection. So, my job going forward was to help make sure not to repeat these circumstances by keeping hydrated and getting plenty of electrolytes.

During the next few weeks, Lorie and I took the early morning train to NY so I could receive an intravenous infusion of chemotherapy as planned. I was quite anxious to resume treatment after a one-week break—especially after seeing reductions in tumor size from the recent CT scan.

On August 22nd, 2017, we finished treatment by early evening and planned on staying in NYC overnight rather than rushing to get home. Since I was hungry for a change, Lorie and I went to the hotel's rooftop bar and enjoyed dinner outside under the stars. It's moments like those that make everything worth it—and I savor every one.

The rescheduled visit by my sister Brandy, husband Mark, and their two boys, Cameron and Chad, went well the past weekend. I haven't made it back to Chicago to see them in a while, and I was amazed by how much Cameron and Chad had grown since I last saw them. It meant a lot to be able to spend some quality time with all of them, and I appreciated their long drive back-and-forth from Illinois to Pennsylvania just to see me.

Knock on wood; I hoped for things to remain calm for a bit. Lorie was going back to work, and our girls were returning to school. It's always a stressful time for them, so it would be nice for my disease to behave for at least a little while.

––––––––––

Living with a terminal cancer diagnosis introduces a fair amount of ambiguity—almost from day one. I've been able to successfully navigate the sea of uncertainties for the past two years with one notable exception: how much time do I have remaining? Or at the very least, how much time remaining where my quality of life allows me to function as a productive member of society?

At the moment, life wasn't horrible. Sure, I suffered side effects from weekly chemotherapy treatment, such as loss of appetite and fatigue. And I lost my hair but saved a ton of money on haircuts and shampoo.

Enduring weekly chemotherapy is made easier given the fact that my tumors have been decreasing in size according to my last few imaging procedures. Precisely what the tumor regression means regarding extending my life is unknown. Published medical literature still suggests that celebrating the New Year isn't a likely event for me. However, every patient is different—and there is one absolute truth in life: no one knows exactly when or how they will die.

In the interim, my greatest challenge was how to keep busy and stay productive during my remaining time—which could be measured in weeks, months, or years. No one knows for sure. Doing some work was very important to me. One of my favorite quotes on the topic is from Stephen Hawking's 2010 interview with ABC News' Diane Sawyer when asked about the best fatherly advice he had given to his children— "...never give up work. Work gives you meaning and purpose and life is empty without it."

My situation is made even more challenging since I really don't know what to expect each day concerning energy or health. For example, I never could have predicted ending up in the hospital on three separate occasions during July and August (including a trip to the ICU). While life has been calm as of late, there is always the chance that something else is lurking around the corner.

There were also financial considerations. We were fortunate that insurance covered the vast majority of my medical expenses. But not being able to work and the loss of income was our biggest financial challenge, as I was the primary breadwinner for the family. Being on social security disability helped, but the monthly payments barely covered our mortgage. Short of winning the lottery, there was no quick financial fix.

As a patient living with cancer, combined with my biotechnology industry background, it became apparent that I possessed unique experience and knowledge. I decided that such patient-centric information could be shared and applied more broadly in health policy planning and decision-making. Through my blog, publishing opinion editorials, media interviews, and more, I planned on keeping busy by increasing awareness of HPV, its link to six cancers, and the need to increase HPV vaccination rates. Where appropriate, I would also lend my voice to advance or oppose health policy.

My new role as an "expert patient" began with filming an interview with Dr. Jon LaPook, the chief medical correspondent for CBS News. It would be included in a future television segment highlighting the recent rise in head/neck cancer in men due to "oral" human HPV. I was also interviewed for local and national media outlets, including the

Philadelphia Inquirer and *National Public Radio (NPR)*. Lastly, I contributed opinion editorials to *BioCentury, NBC Think*, and *STAT News*.

I felt productive and busy.

———

It was July 2017 when I started my third line of treatment (carboplatin and paclitaxel). Things weren't going great at the time. I remember thinking that I wouldn't make it until my 49th birthday in November. I had two chest tubes to manage the buildup of fluid in the pleural lining of my left lung. My tumors were slowly growing with each CT scan. Additionally, I had an IVC filter put in to manage clots since blood thinners had caused bleeding issues. I was a mess and in-and-out of the hospital constantly.

On November 30th, 2017, however, I received the results of my third consecutive CT scan since starting chemotherapy. The results were quite encouraging, as many of the tumors continued to shrink compared with my prior imaging procedure in August. Importantly, there weren't any new sites of cancer spread.

It looks as though cancer continues to respond to the treatment, which is excellent news. In a perfect world, one would like to see all the tumors disappear entirely. That would, however, be highly unusual so I will gladly accept serial decreases in the tumors from period-to-period.

My experience shows the perils of trying to answer the question every cancer patient wants to know: How much more time do I have left? It doesn't stop us from asking physicians, but as a dear friend consistently points out to me—you have to live in the moment and enjoy every day. Much easier said than done, but sage advice nonetheless.

I can't help but wonder if Humphrey, now an 8-month old puppy, is a good luck charm? We got him about a month before I started chemo treatment and things have been going relatively well since then. Not that we need another reason to love him. He's such a clown, always making us laugh and smile. Of course, we love all of our other pets, but there's just something about Humphrey that makes him unique. At the very least, he's a great therapy dog for me.

Responding with compassion and empathy, Humphrey has in many ways been my savior. I rave about him to everyone who listens. Photographs of Humphrey occupy an unusually large portion of my social media outlets. He loves and serves without expecting anything in return. Of course, a long walk or tennis ball is always welcome.

Call it divine intervention, destiny, fate, karma, or whatever, but I believe that Humphrey came into our lives for a reason. Napping next to me, or more likely on top of me, he's a constant source of comfort. Humphrey is also a good motivator. Staring at me with those big, round eyes and tail wagging—he knows how to prod me into getting off the couch and going for a walk.

———————

December 5th, 2017, marked the beginning of cycle number six for my third-line chemotherapy treatment. Having received five cycles over the past five months, my blood counts are slower to recover—particularly my white blood cells. As a result, Dr. Pfister modified the treatment to forgo the third week of chemo since that is usually about the time that my white blood cells are on the low side. In other words, the most recent two cycles of treatment have been "two weeks on, two weeks off" meaning that I get two chemotherapeutics (carboplatin and paclitaxel) on week one, only paclitaxel on week two, and then a two-week break during weeks three and four before starting the cycle over again.

Considering that the two recent cycles have been reduced regarding the total amount of chemo I'm receiving, it is encouraging to see that each CT scan still shows decreases in the size of some tumors. For example, take the largest tumor (on my spleen) that initially measured 6.4 cm on its longest axis and 6.0 cm on its shortest axis back in early January 2017. Since starting third-line chemo over the summer, those dimensions have decreased on each subsequent CT scan: 5.4 x

4.8 cm, 3.2 x 2.6 cm and most recently 2.9 x 2.0 cm. Many other nodules in my lungs and abdomen are also now 1 cm x 1 cm or smaller.

But just exactly how unusual or encouraging was all of this? During the MSKCC appointment, I gathered that the general expectation would have been decreased disease from the first treatment cycle, perhaps stable disease on the second cycle and then possibly progressive disease on the third or later cycles. Bottom line: my cancer continued to decrease across all three recent scans, which is better than normally expected.

I'm happy with the results and incredibly thankful that I received strong encouragement to give chemotherapy another chance. And it's not just about tumors shrinking, there have also been meaningful improvements in my quality of life. For instance, at the start of chemotherapy, I had not one but two chest tubes placed to help reduce fluid around my left lung. Both have since been removed, as the fluid buildup is gone. Associated side effects with the fluid, such as coughing and difficulty breathing have also disappeared. Oh, and it is a lot easier to shower without wrapping your chest and abdomen in plastic wrap each time to avoid water getting into the tubes!

I'm a curious person by nature and seeking potential answers as to "why" my disease is responding a bit better than expected to the current chemo regimen. As a long-time champion of immunotherapy, I can't help but wonder about my prior second-line therapy with M7824, an experimental bispecific fully human antibody designed to simultaneously block two immuno-inhibitory pathways (both PD-L1 and TGF-β) that are commonly used by cancer cells to evade the immune system. The aim of this investigational drug is to control tumor growth by restoring and enhancing anti-tumor immune responses.

While receiving M7824 at the NIH as a participant in their Phase I trial, results from biopsies of both my tumor and pleural fluid provided evidence of immune system activation in the vicinity of the tumor, indicating that the experimental agent M7824 was performing as designed.

It's entirely possible that based on the substantial tumor burden in my body, the immune system activation resulting from M7824 might not have been able to overpower the disease. However, with my tumor burden now having decreased substantially through subsequent chemotherapy, I can't help but wonder if M7824 could be playing a role in my ongoing disease improvement.

———

In early January 2018, I had one of my periodic CT scans to determine if my cancer is regressing (good), progressing (bad), or unchanged. The days preceding these imaging sessions are often very difficult for many other cancer patients and me.

Stressing about the results won't change the outcome, but that doesn't stop me from mentally exploring all of the various scenarios. There's even a term for it—scanxiety—coined by fellow cancer survivors.

I find that writing a cancer blog helps keep my mind occupied during periods of scanxiety. Even when I am writing about my disease, the process of organizing my thoughts or researching a topic online is a welcome distraction that helps me pass the time.

Blogs and participation in other online patient forums also make the experiences of cancer illness publicly visible, provide alternative voices to that of the medical expertise, and challenge the traditional patient-doctor relations.[19] What a remarkable era for patient advocacy.

Among the blogs about fashion, food, home design, travel, and others, numerous blogs about severe disease and dying have appeared in recent years. So, one morning, I decided to Google "terminal cancer blogs" to research the writings of other cancer patients. I was looking for common themes among the multitude of cancers, not just my particular diagnosis. I was also generally curious how many "other" bloggers there were like me.

The exercise started innocently enough. Within 0.54 seconds, Google informed me of the approximate 580,000 search results. I clicked on the title of the first one that caught my eye—"Terminally Fabulous." With a positive name like that, I hoped to find an inspirational blog. And I did.

Suddenly, I was engrossed in the life of Lisa Magill, a Brisbane, Australia woman who started her Terminally Fabulous blog in February 2016, three years after being diagnosed with an incurable rare form of stomach cancer at the age of 30. Ominously, the first thing I noticed upon visiting her blog was that the most recent post was from nearly a year ago. Only by following the link to the Terminally Fabulous page on Facebook did I learn that Lisa succumbed to her disease in early March 2017 at the age of 34.

Reading previous entries on Terminally Fabulous, I appreciated Lisa's writing—full of humor, brutal honesty, and courage. In one entry, she referenced Emma Betts, a friend, cancer survivor and inspirational fellow blogger. Through her Dear Melanoma blog, Emma (like Lisa) shared her cancer journey to help educate others about the importance of cancer awareness and protection methods needed to help prevent melanoma. My heart sunk a little more profoundly after reading the opening text of the Dear Melanoma blog: "Hi, I'm Leon, Emma's dad. By now I'm sure you've heard that Emma passed away in April 2017." She was 25.

After visiting several more terminal cancer blogs from my search results, including Darn Good Lemonade, Anna Swabey: Inside My Head, Tina's Journey, Cancer in Context by

Debra Sherman and others, the grim common theme became clear: Terminal cancer indicates a disease that will progress until death with near absolute certainty.

Of course, there are always exceptions. I still "hope" to be one. But what I learned is that more and more terminal cancer patients are placing their most private, personal journeys in this public and impersonal domain we call the Internet. Reading these brave stories and embracing the author's vulnerability serves to remind us all that our time on this planet is limited. Some even provide inspiration to lead happy and more meaningful lives as a result.

I believe that blogging about life with a terminal illness can offer unique insights into how it is to live with cancer and to face the final phase of life. Hidden away and sequestered, removed from everyday experience, death has made a mediated return to the public sphere through digital and networked media.[20]

The results of my CT scan were favorable. There were no new sites of disease and the existing tumors stayed about the same size from the prior scan. Growth in the current tumors or new sites of disease would indicate disease progression and likely necessitate switching therapies.

It started with a runny nose and sneezing last weekend. Then came a cough and a mild fever that never went above 99.7 Fahrenheit—that is until the following Wednesday, February 7th, 2018. A brief telephone discussion with the doctor on call late that evening confirmed that a trip to MSKCC's urgent care facility was in order.

Following my latest round of chemotherapy, a fever of 100.4 Fahrenheit or higher is disconcerting. It could signal that I'm neutropenic—running dangerously low on a type of white blood cell (neutrophils) that serve as the body's primary defense against acute bacterial and certain fungal infections. The chemotherapy I've been receiving can reduce the number of neutrophils circulating in the blood. Alternatively, a fever could be associated with the flu, which is particularly dangerous this season and breaking records.

Lorie and I started packing for an overnight stay at the MSKCC "bed and breakfast" as we like to call it. Before heading out, I hugged each of our dogs—*just in case.* Unfortunately, that simple action set into motion a rush of feelings and steady stream of tears down my cheeks. I was a total mess by the time Lorie backed the car out from the garage. Rosie and Megan weren't home at the time, which in retrospect was probably best.

At first, I failed to appreciate why Lorie attempted to set a new land speed record for shortest travel time between Bucks County, PA and New York City. Then, I remembered how I narrowly missed having a tachycardia event (abnormally fast heart rate) on the New Jersey Turnpike during our last trip to MSKCC's urgent care facility in August 2017 when I ended up in the ICU.

Upon arrival at urgent care just before midnight, a series of tests were ordered—blood work, urine, chest x-ray, and nasal swab to test for influenza. The blood work came back first and my absolute neutrophil count (ANC) was 800 cells per microliter of blood. With an ANC below 1,000 cells per microliter of blood, the risk of infection increases. Combined with my fever, the medical team informed me that I was going to be admitted to the hospital and given a broad spectrum, intravenous antibiotic Zosyn® (piperacillin and tazobactam).

One by one, the other test results came back normal— that is until the nasal swab revealed I was positive for Influenza B. Influenza A and B are the two main types that routinely spread in humans and cause seasonal flu epidemics. Fortunately, I had received a flu shot this season, as this can help reduce the severity of the virus.

Alas, being hospitalized ended the longest "uneventful" streak of my cancer experience. But for six glorious months, living with cancer was relatively dull and boring. And it was wonderful.

With the source of my fever identified as the flu, I was prescribed Tamiflu® (oseltamivir phosphate) and the general plan was to release me from the hospital as soon as my ANC returned to 1,000 or higher. My prior chemotherapy was given on January 30th, so its adverse effect on my blood counts should be diminishing. Patients often have their lowest number (called a nadir) and highest risk of infection around 7 to 10 days after the start of chemotherapy.

However, my next ANC count was 400. When ANC falls below 500 cells per microliter (severe neutropenia), the risk of infection increases significantly. Accordingly, my stay at the bed and breakfast was extended.

By Friday, my ANC rebounded slightly to 700. Heading in the right direction, but still below the 1,000-level needed for my release home. I felt much better than when I was admitted, which was frustrating. In fact, the fever went away as did a runny nose, sneezing, and coughing.

A repeat blood test was scheduled for very early Saturday morning, with the expectation that my ANC would finally rise above 1,000 and we'd be sent home. Or so I hoped. But the test results showed a slight decrease from the prior day to 600.

I was then given a shot of Neupogen® (filgrastim), which works like a natural protein in your body to promote the growth of new white blood cells. Interestingly, Neupogen was among the very first biotechnology products that I learned about during my introduction to the sector in the late 1990s. It was approved by the FDA back in 1991.

Shortly after the Neupogen injection, my ANC improved and I was released from the hospital.

———————

Finally. The type of day that begs you to go outdoors. Sunny and warm, with just the hint of a breeze. Time to go outside and shake the winter blues. *Just a walk; no purpose this time.*

I didn't need to ask our three dogs if they were interested. As soon as I grabbed a leash, they all swarmed me like I was holding leftover steak. I used to be able to manage two at a time for a walk, but not anymore. Three guesses as to which pup got to go first.

For the past few years, I've received three separate cancer treatments with little reprieve from many of the associated toxicities. On March 6th, 2018, I finished my ninth cycle of therapy—a combination of two chemotherapeutics (carboplatin and paclitaxel). The treatment has significantly reduced the size of tumors in my lungs and spleen, but they have not entirely gone away. My two chest tubes were removed as the fluid in my lung cleared. My heart rate has been stable since starting medication. I celebrated my family's birthdays, observed several holidays, welcomed the New Year, and even commemorated our 26th wedding anniversary in March. I have been given additional precious time.

Following my last cycle of chemo, I had my periodic CT scan to assess whether the cancer is progressing, regressing, or continuing to remain stable. The positive results, which came on March 21st, 2018, showed no new metastases (the spread of cancer) and unchanged disease in my spleen and lungs since my last CT scan on January 19th, 2018.

At the encouragement of Dr. Pfister, and after a great deal of consideration, I decided to take a well-deserved break from treatment. I hope that this pause in therapy helps me heal both physically and mentally. Perhaps it will even allow me to travel and hike.

In a few months, I'll have another CT scan to see how my cancer behaved during the break. I'm cautiously optimistic that my disease will remain stable or perhaps progress slightly, although anything is possible. I still recall how quickly I went from "no evidence of disease" to the progression of disease in both lungs and spleen.

I'm proud of everything that I've accomplished since my initial diagnosis back in December 2015. This includes significantly raising awareness of HPV, its link to six cancers, and the need for increased HPV vaccination through numerous media articles, radio interviews, television appearances, and more than 80 blog posts.

I believe that my current "walk with purpose" as an expert patient is far from finished. But with spring and summer around the corner—I want to get outside, travel, and enjoy life without being hampered by the deleterious effects of chemotherapy.

Regardless of what happens in the future, reflecting on my life I'm simply amazed at how the paths and connections intertwined to lead me to this final destination. I'm acutely aware and appreciative of the advantages that I've had in navigating treatment options. That is why I decided to "pay it forward" by continuing my walk to the very end.

Before cancer, I was wandering aimlessly with no real goal in life other than a desire for material wealth. Now I am someone with a deep motivation, a purpose in life, a definite direction, and an overpowering conviction that there will be a reward at the end of it all.

I hope that I will be around to see the many miracles of science that I believe are close at hand in battling numerous diseases, including my own. If not, however, I had a truly amazing life. I will rest easy knowing that my family and future generations may be helped by the efforts of the biotechnology industry and feel honored to have played even a tiny role as an industry executive and advocate for the sector. Also, I hope that the knowledge gained through my participation in clinical studies will benefit many others.

My story may be unique in some ways, but it is also universal and will resonate, hopefully, for many people fighting against cancer and other diseases.

About the Author

Michael D. Becker

Biotech entrepreneur, author and expert patient

Michael Becker was first diagnosed with Stage IV oropharyngeal (head and neck) cancer caused by the human papillomavirus (HPV) in December 2015. After undergoing aggressive chemoradiation treatment, he was cancer-free for six months. Then, in December 2016, doctors discovered distant metastasis in both of his lungs. Recurrence of this disease is often lethal—no effective treatment exists.

Mr. Becker is a former C-level industry executive with over 25 years of life sciences experience, including serving as CEO for two public biotechnology companies working in the treatment and diagnosis of cancer. During his tenure at New Jersey-based Cytogen Corporation, Mr. Becker raised more than $130 million in new capital through both public offerings and private placements and in-licensed Caphosol©, a topical, oral agent and prescription medical device commercialized for the treatment of oral mucositis and xerostomia.

He is the founder and president of MDB Communications LLC, a provider of investor relations, public relations, and digital media services to the biotechnology industry.

Michael Becker completed coursework in Political Science at DePaul University and received an Associate of Science Degree from the Art Institute of Pittsburgh.

References

[1] Gleeson, Michael, Amanda Herbert, and Aurelia Richards. "Management of Lateral Neck Masses in Adults." BMJ⬚: British Medical Journal 320.7248 (2000): 1521–1524. Print.

[2] Zoumalan, R A et al. "Lymph Node Central Necrosis on Computed Tomography as Predictor of Extracapsular Spread in Metastatic Head and Neck Squamous Cell Carcinoma: Pilot Study." The Journal of laryngology and otology 124.12 (2010): 1284–1288. PMC. Web. 4 Apr. 2018.

[3] Dasari, Shaloam, and Paul Bernard Tchounwou. "Cisplatin in Cancer Therapy: Molecular Mechanisms of Action." European journal of pharmacology 0 (2014): 364–378. PMC. Web. 4 Apr. 2018.

[4] Bruce R. Schatz and Joseph B. Hardin. "NCSA Mosaic and the World Wide Web: Global Hypermedia Protocols for the Internet." Science 12 Aug. 1994: 895-901.

[5] "A Brief History of NSF and the Internet." National Science Foundation. 13 Aug. 2003. Web. 6 Apr. 2018.

[6] "Number of internet users worldwide from 2005 to 2017." Statista. Jul. 2017. Web. 6 Apr. 2018.

[7] Sy Harding. "Are We In Another 1990s Style Super Bull Market?" Forbes. 5 Dec. 2014. Web. 6 Apr. 2018.

[8] Derr, Aaron. "Colorado's Great 14ers." Boys' Life, vol. 107, no. 6, Boy Scouts of America, June 2017, p. 25.

[9] Transferable Priority Review Vouchers fo. https://www.neurotechindustry.org/transferable-priority-review-vouchers-fo#!

[10] Timeline: Key events in financial crisis - USA TODAY. https://www.usatoday.com/story/money/business/2013/09/08/chronology-2008-financial-crisis-lehman/2779515/

[11] Dendreon's Scientific Breakthrough Fails To Sell - yahoo.com. https://www.yahoo.com/news/dendreons-scientific-breakthrough-fails-sell-134902329.html

[12] Vera-Llonch, M., Oster, G., Hagiwara, M. and Sonis, S. (2006), Oral mucositis in patients undergoing radiation treatment for head and neck carcinoma. Cancer, 106: 329-336.

[13] Papas AS, Clark RE, Martuscelli G, O'Loughlin KT, Johansen E, Miller KB. (2003), A prospective, randomized trial for the prevention of mucositis in patients undergoing hematopoietic stem cell transplantation. Bone Marrow Transplant, 31(8):705-12.

[14] Bhat, Zeenat Yousuf et al. "Understanding the Risk Factors and Long-Term Consequences of Cisplatin-Associated Acute Kidney Injury: An Observational Cohort Study." Ed. Partha Mukhopadhyay. PLoS ONE 10.11 (2015): e0142225. PMC. Web. 24 Apr. 2018.

[15] Goenka, Anuj et al. "Long-Term Regional Control in the Observed Neck Following Definitive Chemoradiation for Node-Positive Oropharyngeal Squamous Cell Cancer." International journal of cancer. Journal international du cancer 133.5 (2013): 1214–1221. PMC. Web. 24 Apr. 2018.

[16] Jemal A, Siegel R, Xu J, Ward E. Cancer statistics, 2010. CA Cancer J Clin. 2010;60:277–300.

[17] Ferlito A, Shaha A, R, Silver C, E, Rinaldo A, Mondin V, Incidence and Sites of Distant Metastases from Head and Neck Cancer. ORL 2001;63:202-207.

[18] Azarbarzin, Mehrdad, Azadeh Malekian, and Fariba Taleghani. "Adolescents' Experiences When Living With a Parent With Cancer: A Qualitative Study." Iranian Red Crescent Medical Journal 18.1 (2016): e26410. PMC. Web. 28 Apr. 2018.

[19] Andersson Y. (2017 Jan 1). Blogs and the Art of Dying: Blogging With, and About, Severe Cancer in Late Modern Swedish Society. Omega (Westport).

[20] Lagerkvist, A. (2013). New Memory Cultures and Death: Existential Security in the Digital Memory Ecology. Thanatos, 2(2), pp. 1-17.

Made in the USA
Lexington, KY
22 May 2018